ESSAYS ON THE FIRST HUNDRED YEARS OF ANÆSTHESIA

TO NAN

who pushed me into this labour of Hercu*l*es in the first place; and who helped, loved, cherished and over-fed me through the joyous and delightful years of its fulfilment;

AND IN MEMORY OF

MY FATHER

who had a cholecystectomy done by a most skilful surgeon, with all the ritual, panoply, safety and security of modern surgery, . . . and died thereafter.

AND IN MEMORY OF

HER FATHER,

to whom exactly the same tragic thing happened.

In the hope that this work may help indirectly towards safer surgery. For the value of history lies in the fact that we learn by it from the mistakes of others. Learning from our own is a slow process.

ESSAYS ON THE FIRST HUNDRED YEARS OF ANÆSTHESIA

by

W. STANLEY SYKES,
M.B.E., M.B., B.Chir. (Cantab.), D.A.

Late Anæsthetist to the General Infirmary at Leeds, to the Hospital for Women and St. James' Hospital, Leeds, to the Leeds Dental Hospital, to the Halifax Royal Infirmary and to the Dewsbury General Hospital

Volume II

WOOD LIBRARY – MUSEUM OF ANESTHESIOLOGY
Sponsored by
AMERICAN SOCIETY OF ANESTHESIOLOGISTS
515 Busse Highway Park Ridge, Illinois 60068

CHURCHILL LIVINGSTONE
Medical Division of Longman Group Limited

Distributed in the United States of America and Canada
by the American Society of Anesthesiologists Inc.,
515 Busse Highway, Park Ridge, Illinois 60068.
Distributed elsewhere throughout the world by Churchill
Livingstone and associated companies, branches and
representatives.

First published 1960
Reprinted 1982

ISBN 0 443 02866 4

Printed in Great Britain by
William Clowes (Beccles) Limited,
Beccles and London

PREFACE

THIS volume, in some of its chapters at any rate, stresses much more than its predecessor, the practical value of history to the anæsthetist.

Two of the reviewers of the first volume said that I had been unkind to the Edinburgh school of medicine. Now reviewers are entitled to say what they like, so I do not resent this in the least. In any case they were very kind to me; but I would like to explain that I have no axe to grind, that I have no prejudice against any particular school, and no reason to prefer any one to another—except that I have the normal love for my own University. I shall be relating in a future Essay how I once criticised it very bitterly—and how I was totally wrong. It was one of the silliest things I ever did.

In Volume I, however, all I did was to collect the evidence as exactly and accurately as I could and contrast it with the outrageous and unfounded claims of some injudicious Edinburgh surgeons of the nineteenth century. The facts and the myth which they built up around them did not correspond in any way, and I said so. I still say so; but that is not my fault. It was the fault of the myth-makers, who ignored altogether the absence of foundations for their legend. If they had stuck to the facts there would have been no criticism from me.

W. STANLEY SYKES.

CONTENTS

PLATES

ILLUSTRATIONS

CHAPTER I

THIRTY-SEVEN LITTLE THINGS WHICH HAVE ALL CAUSED DEATH

"Experience is the best of schoolmasters, only the school fees are heavy."
—THOMAS CARLYLE.

IN this essay I propose to deal with certain assorted and somewhat bizarre methods of killing patients, apart from the obvious and prosaic ones. Nobody will have been so unfortunate as to meet them all personally, so some, at least, may be new to many people. Others of course are well known in theory, even to those who have been lucky enough or skilful enough to avoid them. One thing is certain—all of them have happened. All have killed, and they are waiting to do the same thing again unless you know about them. Therein lies the value of history.

Clover's chloroform apparatus was designed to make an overdose of chloroform absolutely impossible. Its main disadvantage was that it was very cumbersome. Even anæsthetists who are familiar with pictures of the whiskered gentleman with an enormous bag slung over his shoulder may not realise that it was not infallible, for it caused at least one death in 1873.[1] It was used on a patient at Broadmoor. A measured dose of chloroform, of 25 minims per 1000 cubic inches (16·387 litres) was injected into the bag, which was nominally of 11,000 cubic inches capacity (180 litres). The bag was then filled with air by means of the bellows provided. As the 25 minims of chloroform produced 28 cubic inches of vapour the mixture in the bag was fixed at 2·8 per cent., which could not be exceeded—in theory. But the patient died. Three weeks later the mystery was solved,[2] when the inhaler was examined by Mr. Clover and the maker, Mr. Coxeter. It was found that the capacity of the bag was only 8400 cubic inches, instead of its reputed 11,000. This meant that the amount of chloroform put in would give a vapour, not of 2·8 per cent. but of 3·66 per cent. The bellows were also stiff from disuse and did not deliver their full quota of air, which no doubt prevented the unduly small capacity of the bag being detected by the number of bellows-strokes required to fill it. It was suggested that the cubic capacities of the bags should be carefully measured and stamped on the bags themselves.

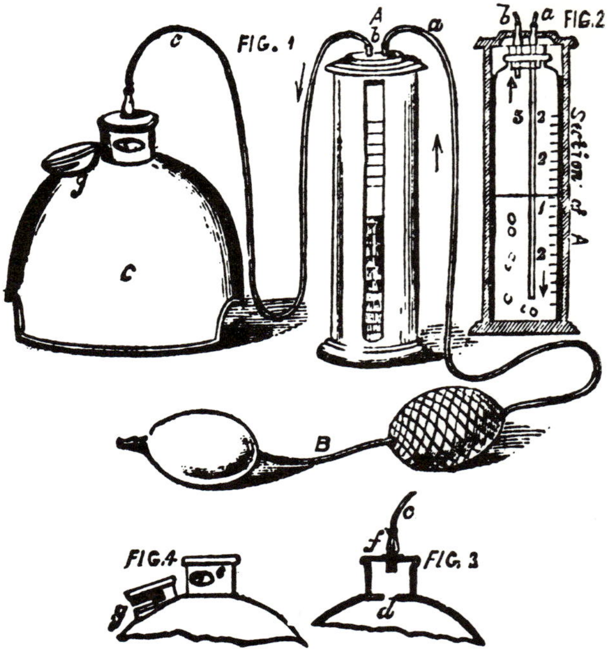

FIG. 1

Medical Times and Gazette, 1867, Nov. 30. 590. F. E. Junker, London. New apparatus for administering narcotic vapours. A glass cylinder holds 2 ounces of fluid. It fits into a velvet-lined stand, which is needed to prevent chloro-methyl boiling in a hot room. The mask C is made of vulcanite. E is an air slot for use with choloroform. G Expiratory valve. Made by Krohne & Sesemann.

This, the original picture of Junker's inhaler, took me over a year to find, after discovering innumerable modifications of it.

In an era when chloroform was practically the only anæsthetic, and before electric lighting came into general use, there were many reports of trouble from the decomposition of chloroform when it was given near the open flame of a candle or gas lamp. K. Wilson[3] gave chloroform to a midwifery case in a small room with three gas jets burning. It caused such violent coughing and gasping for breath that forceps could not be applied, and the operation was concluded under ether. Professor Zweifel had seven deaths out of nine laparotomies done under chloroform by gas light. Mey, of Herne, Westphalia, repaired a gunshot wound of the abdomen, evidently a complicated one, for it took four hours. One of the nurses died two days later. Iterson[4] had had the same sort of trouble ten years earlier. In 1894[5] the *Lancet*, on receiving another cry of distress, explained that phosgene was produced when chloroform was decomposed in this way.

$$2CHCl_3 + O_2 = 2\ COCl_2 + 2HCl.$$

In 1906 John T. Bouchier-Hayes,[6] quoting Dawbarn, advised dipping handkerchiefs in ammonia and hanging them up near the lights. Ammonium chloride is formed at once and the room freed from irritant gases.

This phenomenon was not always fatal, but it has killed people. No doubt the severity of its effects would depend on the size of the room, its ventilation, the length of the operation and the distance from the chloroform mask to the gas jet. At the best it must have been extremely unpleasant. The small room with open flames in it must have presented a difficult problem. You could only choose between poisoning everybody with phosgene or blowing them up with an ether explosion.

Another prolific source of death was the Junker's inhaler. In its original form[7] it was not fitted with any safeguard against connecting up the tubes wrongly, which must have happened a great many times. The frequent and vicious custom of allotting the anæsthetic to anybody, however junior and inexperienced, made this quite certain. A student, given a Junker's inhaler which he had never seen before and told to pump air through it, would naturally do so, quite regardless of whether the bulb was attached to the proper tube, and quite unaware of the disastrous results if it were not. Even more experienced persons were not infallible. As late as 1917, fifty years after the introduction of the method and twenty-five years after a perfectly safe apparatus was available, R. W. Lloyd[8] reported that he had fallen into this trap. The whole of the liquid chloroform was pumped into the patient. He was lucky, for the patient recovered after artificial respiration and tracheotomy. Rickard W. Lloyd was born in 1859 and qualified in 1880. He was anæsthetist to the West London Hospital. He died on April 24th, 1933.

Nor were the original Junker and its early successors safe if they were tilted or shaken. Liquid chloroform could, and did, pass over under these conditions.

The first modification of the original Junker was made by Joseph Mills, chloroformist to St. Bartholomew's Hospital, in 1878.[9] He replaced the facepiece by a flexible metal tube, which could be inserted into the nose or mouth. This alteration, though it did not increase its safety, except possibly by lessening the risk of overdose, enabled full

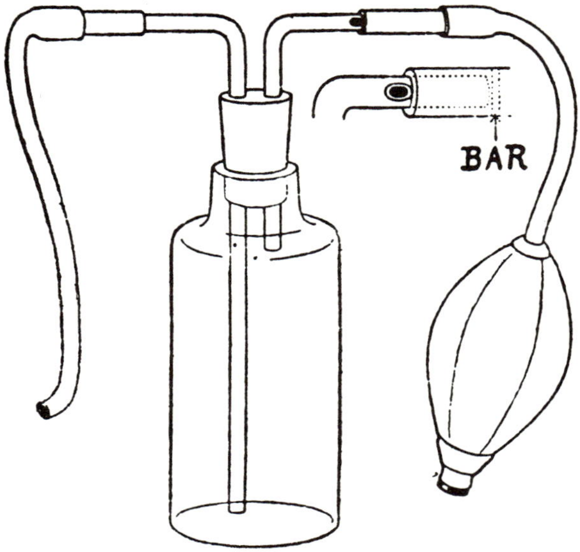

FIG. 2

Lancet, 1919, Nov. 15. 880. E. L. Kennaway. Safety chloroform inhaler. Made by Maw. Shown wrongly put together. The bar across the lumen of the tube ensures that the hole is left open. The facepiece tube has no bar, so that it can cover the hole.

advantage to be taken of the convenience of the vapour method in operations in which any mask was in the way of the surgeon.

In 1883 Krohne and Sesemann[10] produced a model with a hook attached, so that the chloroformist could hang the apparatus on one of his button holes. It also had a bulb which delivered a measured quantity of air, which in turn vapourised a known quantity of chloroform.

Dudley Buxton[11] added a filling funnel and a foot bellows, both of which increased its convenience but not its safety. Krohne and Sesemann[12] then brought out their facepiece with a hinged feather indicator over the expiratory valve. This model also had the flexible metal tube as an alternative to the facepiece.

But these were trivialities. The first real important advance in safety came from Frederic Hewitt in 1892.[13] He stated that deaths had occurred through the tubes being wrongly connected and also through hanging the apparatus on the coat, which led to variations in the level of the liquid chloroform. His new model hung round the anæsthetist's neck, and the two tubes were of different sizes, one inside the other.

Two months later Carter Braine,[14] having personally seen a death from tilting the inhaler, produced yet another design which made both these mistakes impossible. His tubes were not interchangeable, and the inhaler was safe in any position. Charles Carter Braine, who died on September 1st, 1937, aged 78, was anæsthetist to Charing Cross Hospital. His father, F. W. Braine, had held the same post before him.

There are plenty of other designs to choose from, but the above will be sufficient. Obviously a great number of people gave serious thought to this problem, but for many years after safety instruments were available the old, dangerous models continued to be used, sometimes disastrously. W. J. Foster,[15] after a fatal case in 1927, destroyed all the valveless inhalers in the hospital, and advised that this should be done everywhere. This particular patient was a boy of 16, who died in 24 hours from oedema of the lungs. The inhaler had been assembled by a corporal in a military hospital. The next year there was another death,[16] and the *Lancet* took the trouble to describe several forms of safety inhalers.

But we have not quite finished with Junker's apparatus yet. C. F. Hadfield[17] reported a death in 1919 in which a Junker, *correctly assembled,* delivered liquid instead of vapour. This, he found, could happen if the vapour exit was too low or if the full two ounces of chloroform were put in and the bulb violently pumped. Nor have we finished with chloroform. In 1931 there was a death from an explosion under chloroform, incredible and impossible as this sounds.[18] A pencil light was in the mouth. The ether bottle of the Shipway's apparatus had been turned off and oxygen was being passed through chloroform. There was an explosion in the patient's mouth and the apparatus blew up. Death took place in five days. Autopsy showed bruising of the pharynx, a tear in the left pyriform fossa and haemorrhages in the epiglottis. Obviously in this case the ether tap was not gas-tight, and the current of oxygen passing it on its way to the chloroform bottle sucked up some ether vapour. It was found that a 4-volt spark would not ignite ether and air, but would ignite ether and oxygen.

Talking of explosions, when I began to construct this essay from a packet of cards taken from my card index, I thought that these disasters would be classified into two groups—those due to sparks from electrical apparatus and those from static electricity. I found that this was an under-estimate. There were really five groups.

The first was, of course, due to sparks from defective lights, switches, or other electrical apparatus, the use of an actual cautery in the presence of an inflammable vapour, and so on. Non-electrical sources of ignition, such as open flames, are not likely to be a problem in a modern operating theatre, but may still be of importance in practice outside hospitals. In the days of candles, oil-lamps and gas jets they were much more frequently dangerous.

Thomas Nunneley of Leeds[19] had two fires in his experimental work in 1849. These were probably two of the earliest ever recorded. One of them arose from inserting a glowing splinter of wood into a jar of oxygen, the other from inspecting a jar of volatile inflammable liquid with a lighted candle.

"Expt. No. 118. A very large and powerful old male cat was put into a jar . . . with a drachm of oleum aethereum, and covered over. It was very late at night, and only one candle left burning. . . . As the light was not very good, in three minutes the cover was removed, and the candle brought near to ascertain the effects; he was seen to be crouched down, soundly asleep; but inadvertently in examining, the candle was brought too near, the vapour became inflamed, and in an instant the whole jar was in a fearful blaze, the cat being completely enveloped in it. The only means to extinguish it was to exclude the air by putting on the cover; this was done; and the flame very soon went out, when the cat was still soundly asleep, not having stirred, being altogether unconscious of the fire. . . ."

J. Mason Warren[20] recorded two fires by 1868, one of them due to a lamp three feet away, the other due to a red hot cautery in the mouth. To come to more modern times, the early Boyle's gas oxygen machines introduced about the end of the First World War were fitted with a small spirit lamp which was hung on the framework with the flame playing on the valve of the nitrous oxide cylinder which was in use at the time. The reason for this was that nitrous oxide, at that period, was not thoroughly dried by the makers and contained enough water vapour to freeze up the valves after flowing for a short time. This spirit lamp never appeared to be a very safe arrangement, considering that an ether bottle was incorporated in the same machine, not very far away from the open flame. To make matters worse, the ether bottle was *above* the level of the lamp. Some people used to put hot water bottles on the neck of the cylinder as a substitute. H. W. Featherstone reported an explosion of a gas bag caused by this spirit lamp in 1931.[21]

The third great cause of explosions, of course, is static or frictional electricity. Sparks from this cause, while common in the dry climate of the United States, are rare in the damp atmosphere of England, but they are not unknown. R. Ironside[22] described one in 1935. Alarming and spectacular though it was, nobody was killed in this particular accident. The anæsthetic trolley had been in use for two and a half hours and was being wheeled into the anæsthetic room to start the next case. There was a violent explosion. Three people were knocked over, the patient fell off the trolley and the whole room was a sheet of flame. The swing doors into the theatre were blown open three times with great bursts of flame. All electrical plugs were found to be in good order, but the humidity in the theatre was very low. There had been complaints of static sparks on several occasions before the explosion happened.

Ironically enough the risk in this country is greater in operating theatres which have been modernised. Steam heated sterilisers were often fitted in a recess in the theatre itself, which kept the air at a constant humidity high enough to be safe. They are now banished to another room, and up goes the explosion risk.

A fourth principle is involved in fires and explosions, this time flameless and sparkless, namely the heat generated by the sudden compression of a gas. G. Ramsey Phillips in 1931[23] reported a fire in an oxygen cylinder valve due to the sudden opening of the cylinder (main) valve with the fine adjustment valve shut. The sudden liberation of high-pressure oxygen compressed the air in the space between the two valves—and something, presumably grease or a washer, caught fire. This is the principle used in the ignition of a Diesel engine. The reducing valve should always be opened first, and great care taken to avoid oil, grease or inflammable washers.

The fifth principle is that of catalytic action. On October 8th, 1925, a boy of 16 broke his jaw in a cycling accident.[24, 25] Ether and oxygen anæsthesia had been in progress for 25 minutes and the operation was practically over. Warm air was being applied from a dental syringe in order to dry the teeth. The lamp for warming the air was six feet away and there were no naked lights nearer. The syringe was not red hot. On the third syringeful of air there was an explosion at the back of the patient's mouth. Acute hæmorrhage ensued followed by death in ten minutes. Rupture of the bronchi and collapse of the lungs were found at post-mortem.

Bernard D. Bolas[26] suggested that the catalytic action of the metal parts of the syringe had caused the ignition. This was an ingenious solution which may very well have been correct; but it must be admitted that this is not certain, for two other explanations were put forward, either of which could have been the cause.

J. N. Loring[27] experimented with a dental hot-air syringe and a spirit lamp. He found that it was possible to pick up a tiny fragment of burning carbon from the wick on the end of the syringe and to carry it some distance with the fragment still burning. Also, by pushing the nozzle of the syringe into the surface of the wick, he could pick up and convey a small drop of burning spirit.

C. F. Hadfield and H. B. Dixon[25] pointed out that ether could burn with a 'cool flame' at a temperature below 190° C., which is 300° C. below visible redness. Normal ignition needs a temperature of 360°C. No definite conclusion was ever reached in this case, as far as I know, but the theory of catalytic action is at least possible.

I am happy to say that I have never seen an anæsthetic explosion. The nearest approach to it was when a gynæcologist came into the anæsthetic room and casually leaned on a 750-gallon ethylene cylinder with a lighted cigarette in his hand! I can remember my squawk of horror to this day. The psychic shock was considerable, but nothing happened. I was using ethylene quite a lot at that time and it was mere chance that the cylinder was turned off.

Before leaving the subject of explosions there are two other causes of death, again due to compressed air, but this time nothing to do with Diesel ignition or ignition of any sort. I have only found one fatality due to the first of these. B. B. Lennon and E. A. Rovenstine,[28] in an eight column article, describe a death from the bursting of the cuff on an endotracheal tube. The 'explosion' here would be so small and so weak that it could happen in many cases without doing any damage.

H. D. Gillies, T. Pomfret Kilner and A. H. McIndoe[29] reported a fatal case of stomach inflation during 'endotracheal' insufflation.

It is an easy transition from these compressed air deaths to another fatality due to oxygen under pressure. This was in no sense of the word an explosion or even an over-distension, but acted in quite a different way—and just as fatally.

Usually with an intermittent flow apparatus overdosage from nitrous oxide need not be feared. As oxygen is a direct and immediate antidote to gas, one has only to press the emergency button to direct a spurt of oxygen into the lungs and resuscitation takes place immediately, so long as gas alone is being used. This is so even if the breathing has stopped altogether, because the oxygen is forced in under pressure, though it is preferable to follow McKesson's advice and anticipate this—"The last breath but one should have plenty of oxygen in it."

There is no risk of damage to the lungs, because it is not possible to

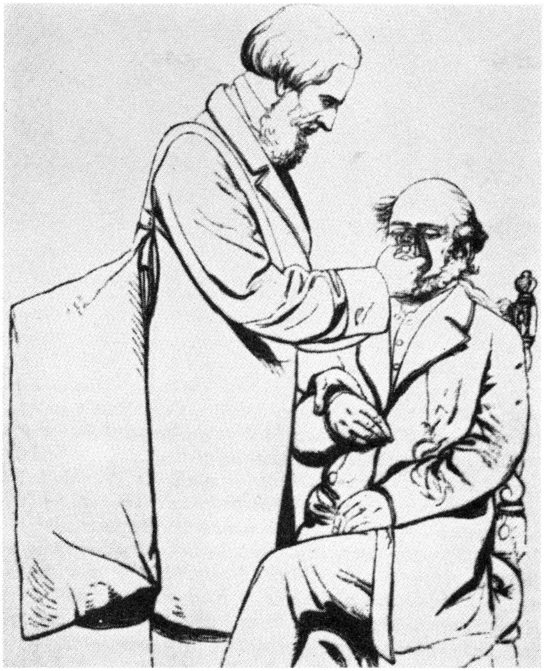

PLATE I

Clover's chloroform apparatus. The large bag slung over the shoulder is lined with goldbeater's skin to make it airtight. The outer covering would no doubt be some thin fabric. Into the bag are injected measured doses of chloroform. The bag is then filled with air by means of a bellows. 20 minims to each 1000 cubic inches capacity would give $2\frac{1}{4}\%$, as 20 minims give rise to 22·5 cubic inches of vapour. 30 minims would give 3·37% and so on. The patient inhaled the mixture from the bag and exhaled it through an expiratory valve. There was, of course, no rebreathing.

From *Chloroform, its action and administration,* by Arthur Ernest Sansom. 1865. London: John Churchill. p. 187.

Sansom was born May 13, 1838, qualified 1859. Became Physician to the London Hospital. Died March 10, 1907. A very good little book. He records 109 deaths from chloroform from 1847 to 1865, a period of 18 years.

Joseph Thomas Clover was born February 28, 1825. He was present at Liston's first operation under ether (Wm. Squire, *Lancet, 1882, Oct. 14. 649.*) Became Resident Medical Officer at University College Hospital, 1848. Then confined his practice to anæsthetics. He gave chloroform to Napoleon III on January 2, 1873, at Chislehurst. Sir Henry Thompson sounded and detected a stone. Lithotrity performed. January 6. Clover anæsthetised him again for another sitting. The Emperor died January 9. Clover signed the post mortem report with five others. He gave an anæsthetic to the Prince of Wales (later Edward VII) in 1877, for an abscess attributed to a hunting injury. He designed a bladder evacuator. He died, age 57, September 27, 1882.

He also gave chloroform to H.R.H. The Princess of Wales, later Queen Alexandra, for the removal of a splint from a rheumatic knee, in 1867.

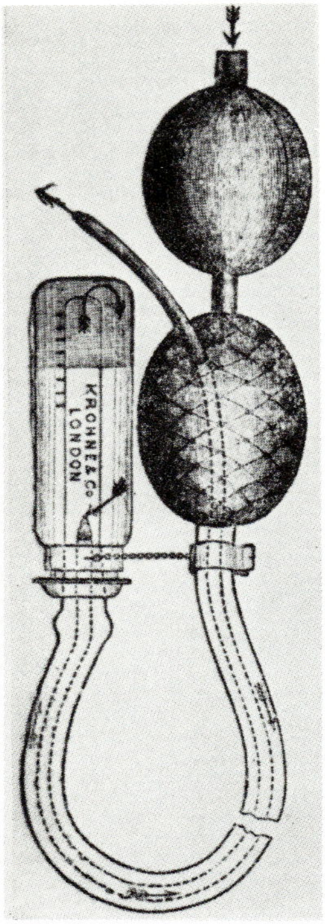

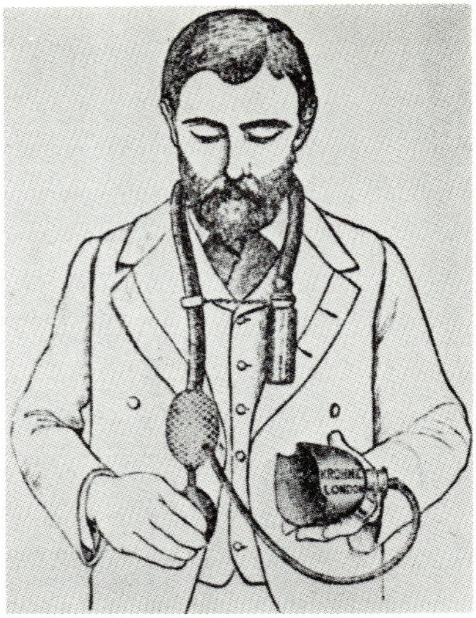

PLATES II and III

Lancet, 1892, Apr. 30. 966. Frederic Hewitt. Modified Junker's inhaler. In the ordinary model deaths have occurred from *a.* connecting the tubes wrongly, and *b.* from hooking the apparatus to the coat, causing tilting. Both these faults can allow liquid chloroform to be delivered instead of vapour. The new model does away with both these defects. It is also convenient without the long flexible tubes.

Made by Krohne & Sesemann.

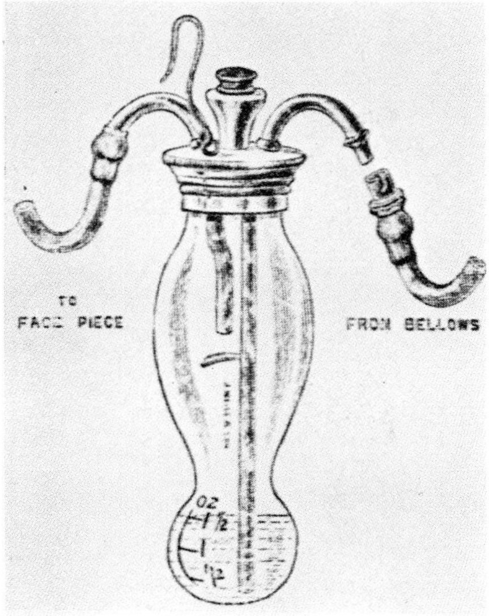

PLATE IV

Briti. med. J. 1892, June 25. 1364. Carter Braine. He had seen death due to liquid chloroform delivered when the bottle was tilted on its side. This model will not deliver liquid in any position, owing to the length of the short tube inside the bottle. Splashing is prevented by the curved guard. The tubes are not interchangeable, so there is no danger from wrong assembly. The level of the liquid must not be above the constriction.

Made by Weiss & Co.

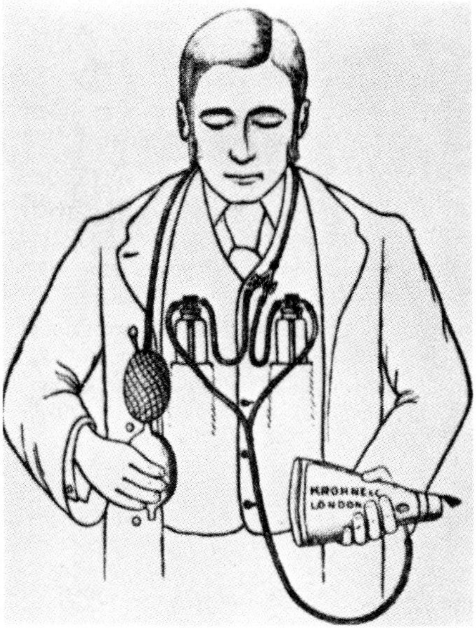

PLATE V

Handbuch der allgemeinem und lokalen Anesthesie. Professor F. L. Dumont. 1903. pp. 234.

Tyrrell's inhaler for mixtures. One bottle is filled with ether and the other with chloroform. A predecessor of the better known Shipway's apparatus.

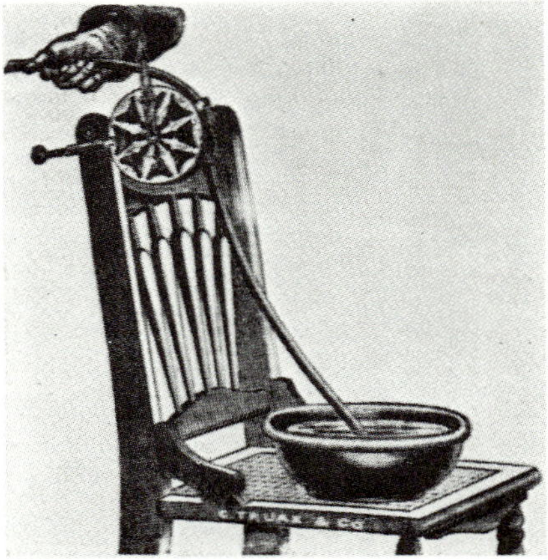

PLATE VI

Brit. med. J., 1888, Sept. 29. 722. The Allen rotary surgical pump. Made by Charles Truax & Co., Chicago. Designed by E. E. Allen of Grand Rapids, Michigan, as a blood transfuser. Can also be used for aspiration, as a stomach pump or for embalming!

A hand driven rotating roller queezes the rubber tube as it revolves.

FIG. 3

Lancet, 1898, June 4. 1555. Krohne & Sesemann's improved Junker's inhalers. They were fitted with the Buxton filling funnel and the feather breathing indicator on the expiratory valve. In their tropical model all the rubber tubing except the exit tubes were replaced by metal tubes. A vulcanite or metal air-pump with a screw stop on its piston rod was used instead of a rubber bulb. Owing to the constrictions in the bottles the chloroform can be regulated to 1/100th minim. The eighth drachm is divided into minims. 18 minims of chloroform will produce deep anæsthesia.

Lancet, 1900, Jan. 13. 132. Clayton Lane, Lt., I.M.S. criticises Krohne's inhaler. Quotes a death in which it had been used. "It cannot be too strongly insisted on that by no merely mechanical means can chloroform be given with safety . . ." " . . . at its best it is little more than an economiser of chloroform." The facepiece may prevent cyanosis being noticed in time.

Lancet, 1900, Jan. 27. 227. James Edmunds. Agrees that no inhaler can supply the user with skill or sense. But it is good to give exact doses. We do not guess the dose of morphia or strychnine, but measure it exactly.

FIG. 4.

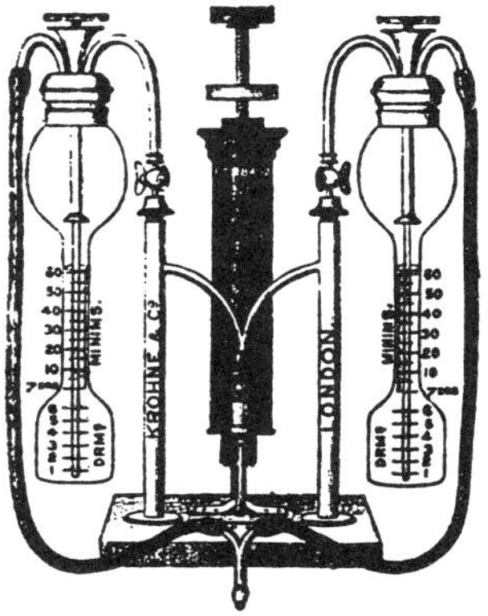

FIG. 5.

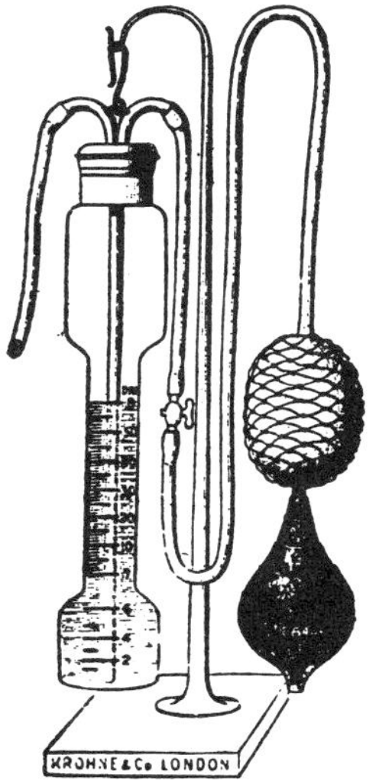

FIG. 3

hold a facepiece on tightly enough to prevent leakage round its rim at a pressure far below a dangerous level. So it seems foolproof. But there is one snag, and only one. Geoffrey Kaye[30] described a death from oxygen used in this way for resuscitation purposes. The patient was having gas and oxygen and became cyanotic. Lung inflation with oxygen was followed, not by immediate recovery, but by deep asphyxia and death. At the post-mortem the bronchial tree was found to be full of vomit, packed closely into it by the pressure of the gas.

Interpretation of this case on the scanty facts given above is somewhat speculative, but I think it admits of only one explanation. Vomiting takes place solely in light anæsthesia and not when the patient is deeply under. This applies to gas as well as any other anæsthetic. (The only exception is the regurgitation of intestinal obstruction, which may occur at any depth.) So, either the cyanosis was due to an unnoticed accumulation of vomit in the first place, and not due to too much nitrous oxide; or somebody was relying on cyanosis as a sign of deep anæsthesia—confusing it with anoxæmia, in fact. Probably the patient was a plethoric person with a large amount of hæmoglobin in his blood, in which case cyanosis would occur easily, perhaps in light anæsthesia, perhaps even before the stage of anæsthesia was reached at all. At this stage he vomited. This was not noticed and the cyanosis was taken to be a sign of deep anæsthesia. If the pharynx had been thoroughly emptied before the inflation all would have been well.

Many lives must have been lost owing to inefficient oxygen apparatus. The old tube and glass funnel method had no effect on the alveolar oxygen content at all, and the fact that the other end of the tube was attached to an oxygen cylinder hardly mattered. (On the other hand disasters began to happen when too-efficient oxygen treatment was developed and used. I refer, of course, to retro-lental fibroplasia in premature babies. This subject is dealt with elsewhere in these essays. It need not detain us here. As far as I know there were no deaths from it. Only permanent blindness. Only!)

Several deaths have taken place owing to other gases being given in mistake for oxygen. In 1940 two patients were killed because carbon dioxide cylinders were substituted for oxygen cylinders.[31] The green code paint of the cylinders had been covered by a coat of black. This happened in a service hospital, and it is a fair assumption that it was due to an inspection 'flap'. Probably some enthusiastic orderly noticed that the green paint looked a bit tatty and proceeded in all innocence to repaint it neatly with the wrong colour, thereby sentencing two of his comrades to death. Or perhaps he thought that all cylinders should be the same colour anyway, especially for an inspection.

Another case occurred four years later.[32] This time it was a nitrous oxide cylinder which was misused. In 1945[33] there was yet another.

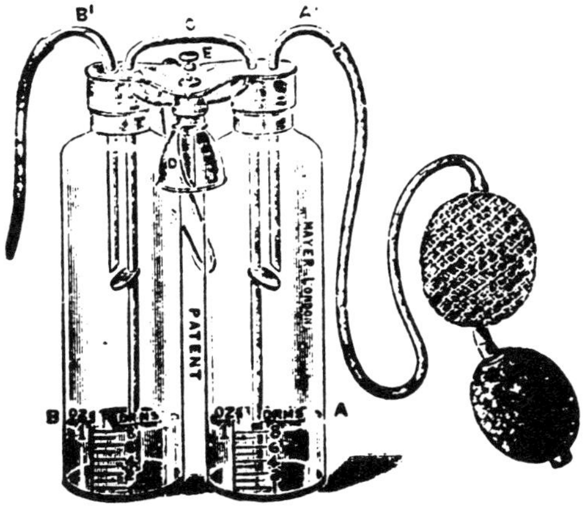

FIG. 4

Lancet, 1928, Dec. 29. 1359. Safety Junker's inhaler. The Chiron, made by Mayer & Phelps. A most ingenious model with two safety devices. Overfilling is impossible with the upside down filling funnel; and the tubes cannot be connected wrongly. Chloroform can be put into either bottle. If it is in the correct one it vapourises correctly and normally; if not, it is merely transferred by the air pressure into the other bottle, where it again vapourises correctly, because this bottle is the opposite way round.

The anæsthetist found the gas machine to be in order, but did not check the cylinders, which were changed by a nurse. The child stopped breathing, was given 'oxygen' and died. The 'oxygen' turned out to be nitrous oxide.

It would seem that it would be worth while to develop a small, compact, quick-acting analyser by which the contents of all cylinders could be rapidly checked before using them. A qualitative test would do, to include all gases.

The *Lancet* said in 1945[34] "these deaths must stop." In fairness the writer pointed out that the anæsthetist generally has no skilled assistance; that distinctive marks and colours may be obliterated and that colours may be indistinguishable in a bad light. Labels may be torn off; the anæsthetist may be tired; he may have been just roused from sleep. No matter, said the *Lancet*, "it must be made impossible to connect a cylinder to any but its appropriate reducing valve and flow-meter."

That sounds uncommonly like sense to me. There are so many mistakes that one can make in anæsthesia—don't forget, I have made most of them myself, and I know—that it seems eminently reasonable if some of them, at least, can be made physically impossible. But a certain and positive safeguard was very slow in making its appearance. Standard colours for different gas cylinders, with different coloured rubber tubing to match were good as far as they went—but they were not infallible.

The earliest reference I have been able to trace, to a mechanical method of making wrong connections impossible was in Lundy's book in 1942.[35] His pictures showed methods of altering the standard cylinders and yokes; it was at least a start. A fully developed pin-index system of eight differently arranged systems of holes drilled in the cylinder valves and correspondingly arranged pins on an adaptor, which can easily be fitted to the yokes, was illustrated in 1954.[36]

Turning, for a change, to a point of trivial importance, it would be interesting to know, as a matter of academic interest, why three different gases are measured for sale in three different units. Why do we buy nitrous oxide by the gallon, oxygen by the cubic foot and carbon dioxide by the pound? Is there any rational explanation of this apparent absurdity?

It is, of course, equally possible to confuse liquids used in anæsthesia as well as gases, though they are easier to distinguish by their weight, their feel and their smell. F. R. Brown[37] once found that he was giving chloroform on an open mask from a drop bottle labelled ether. In this case the error was detected before any harm was done, but I have no doubt whatever that similar mistakes have caused death. Brown suggested the compulsory addition of a harmless red dye to all chloroform. A week later C. J. Massey Dawkins[38] pointed out that Duncan Flockhart of Edinburgh had produced a red chloroform for the last ten years. But chloroform is made by many firms, and there was no uniformity.

Trilene, of course, has been safeguarded by an artificial blue colour ever since its introduction, but then it is made exclusively by one firm. The makers of trilene did what they could to make it safe by its distinctive colour, but this drug had another potential danger which was not foreseen until it had killed several patients. Nobody could be blamed for this. To have predicted this particular danger would have required almost superhuman foresight.

Trichlorethylene was first investigated in this country in 1941,[39] after it had been brought to the notice of the profession by Mr. C. Chalmers of Muswell Hill. It had been known chemically since 1864; it had been used in the treatment of trigeminal neuralgia, and it had caused industrial poisoning when employed as a degreasing agent. It had been used as an anæsthetic as early as 1935, but this was not generally known.

By the time it became popular soda lime absorption had been in general use for nearly ten years. Cyclopropane was responsible for this; being an expensive gas it had to be given in a closed circuit for economy, and so arose the custom of using soda lime with ether or nitrous oxide, when it was not strictly necessary. Most machines were fitted with an absorber of some kind or other and all the then known anæsthetics could be given equally well with or without it. It made no difference to their safety. And so, when trilene was new nobody thought of possible danger —until it happened.

About three years after its introduction J. H. Humphrey and Margaret McClelland[40] reported a new and hitherto unknown syndrome. They had had 13 cases of cranial nerve palsies following general anæsthesia. In 9 of them the palsies were accompanied by herpes. There were 2 deaths in the series. It was found that trichorethylene, used in conjunction with soda lime, combined with it to form dichloroacetylene, a poisonous substance. S. Carden, in the same issue of the journal,[41] also pointed out this danger. The solution of this problem was made more difficult by the fact that some of the palsies occurred in patients who had had no trichlorethylene, which tended to put the investigators off the scent. But it was found that soda lime, once contaminated by trilene and its resultant dichloroacetylene, retained its toxic qualities and could give rise to this form of poisoning even in patients who had had other anæsthetics only, provided that the same soda lime was in use.

The manufacturers reacted with commendable speed to this news. Three weeks later[42] they stated that a warning notice about the use of their product with soda lime now appeared on all packages containing it.

Another instance in which a firm of manufacturing chemists were compelled to take action—not so quickly in this case—was simply and solely due to a trade name. This name caused three deaths, to my knowledge. On such a trivial matter of nomenclature does life depend. Nupercaine, which I believe was always its name in the United States, was known in England as percaine until 1942. I could never understand why these foolish multiplications of unnecessary names are so popular, except on the general principle that business men are usually extremely unbusinesslike.

The short name percaine could easily be confused, either in speech or writing, with procaine, which, of course, is generally used in solutions about ten times as strong. In 1937 a death occurred in Lancashire[43] due to this very confusion. This time it was for local injection only, but 1 per cent. percaine, supplied instead of the 1 per cent. procaine asked for, was injected and the injection was followed by death. The next fatality was at Bournemouth two and a half years later.[44] Three years after this yet another death happened in Oxfordshire.[45] The *Lancet* said that they had hoped at the time of the Bournemouth disaster that the manufacturers would change the name to the American name nupercaine, which was not nearly so likely to be confused. The firm's attitude had been, however, that their name percaine was registered in 1918, whereas the term procaine was not adopted by the British Pharmacopoeia until 1932. Therefore, the firm argued, the official name should be changed.

Fortunately a month later[46] the firm in question had the good sense not to allow such a dangerous situation to continue because of a trivial and unimportant point, and the name percaine was dropped. In future it was nupercaine in this country as well as in America. This addition of two letters to a trade name had been bought at the cost of three lives.

Another source of danger had arisen, involving the use of the same drug; convulsions were reported after its use. There were three cases, one of which died.[47] In the fatal case the drug was not used from an ampoule, but as bulk solution from a 150 cc. flask. It was found afterwards that the solution had evaporated, through prolonged or repeated boiling, from its original volume to just under 100 cc., which of course meant that a considerable overdose was being given when this powerful agent was dispensed by volume. Of the two non-fatal cases one of them was feverish and jaundiced and the other had ovarian cysts of a total weight of about 39 lb. Her true weight was thus considerably less than was realised, with the result that she got a relative overdose.

Nor were the names of drugs the only source of confusion. An anæsthetist once asked for a point one per cent. solution of decicaine.[48] He was given the right drug, but a one per cent. solution. He used it and the patient died. Ten times the dose simply because the word 'point' in the verbal instructions was ignored. He was found not guilty of manslaughter at the subsequent trial. Perhaps Lord Randolph Churchill, Sir Winston's father, had something when he grumbled about the "damned dots" in a

Budget statement. If the decimal system has its dangers, so also has the old apothecary's system. A legal action[49] followed the death of a patient who had been ordered 6 drachms of paraldehyde per rectum as pre-operative medication. The nurse, mistaking the sign ʒ for ℥, gave her six ounces. And so an innocuous pre-medication was multiplied by eight and became a permanent and final euthanasia. It appears, then, that no system of measurement is foolproof. The only solution appears to be the method adopted when writing cheques—all doses to be written both in words and figures. Human lives are surely worth nearly as much as money.

Infection after spinal injections has also caused death on more than one occasion. An epidemic of this infection took place in Sheffield[50] and was reported by H. J. Barrie. Out of 96 patients operated upon under spinal anæsthesia in one particular theatre 11 cases became infected, one of which died. Light percaine solution was used. Suspicion fell upon a cold-water Berkefeld filter, the water from which, presumed to be sterile, was used to rinse the spinal needles and syringes, which had been kept in formalin vapour. It was never actually proved that the filter was the cause, but the epidemic stopped when it ceased to be used.

A year later suspicion fell upon another source of infection. This time it was a war-time makeshift which was at fault. C. Langton Hewer and Lawrence P. Garrod[51] reported that there had been an increase of meningeal infection after spinal anæsthesia. They attributed it to the war-time ampoules, which carried paper labels, instead of having the lettering etched into the glass. Bacteria could be grown from these ampoules after immersion in spirit for half an hour. The authors recommended that they should never be put into a bowl with the sterile needles and syringes. They should be regarded as contaminated, on the outside at least, and held in a sterile towel.

Frankis T. Evans[52] reported two fatal cases of infection from spinal anæsthesia and detailed the necessary precautions to minimise the risk. All syringes and needles should be boiled for five minutes, kept in spirit and used only for spinals. Ampoules should be stored in biniodide and handled wrapped in gauze. Only ampoules should be used, and never bulk solution. Gloves to be worn and spirit and iodine used for skin preparation. An introducer should always be used to prepare the way for the needle, to avoid carrying in skin infection. The needle shafts must not be touched at all. The trolley should be freshly laid out, and no large bottles of water or other liquids used. These always become contaminated.

Harold Dodd[53] gave some very concise instructions for avoiding this disastrous calamity. Boil everything and lay out dry. Towel adequately and wash up thoroughly. W. G. Mills advised boiling the syringe and needle just before use, and washing them out with the anæsthetic solution to be used. The needle should be held in a gauze swab and the skin puncture made with any large needle, *not* the one to be used for the injection, thus preventing a lump of epidermis of doubtful sterility being impaled on the point of the spinal needle.[54]

D. W. C. Northfield[55] attacked the problem in an entirely different and rather startling way. He stated that wet hands or wet gloves always contaminated the needle by liquid running on to it. Therefore *do not* wash up at all, but use a rigid no-touch technique. Hold the needle in a sterile towel. This method, he said, was always used in the neuro-surgical unit in which he worked, for all their lumbar punctures.

Most of the spinals and locals which I have given were given in a prisoner-of-war hospital in Germany. We had a good operating theatre, but equipment was somewhat scanty. The pressure on the German Army Medical Stores must have been enormous, even allowing for all the equipment that was captured. As we only had one steriliser for all purposes, spinal syringes and needles could not be boiled in it because it contained the usual rust-preventing alkali. So my syringes and needles had to be boiled separately in a Red Cross milk-powder tin. It didn't look quite as impressive as a chromium plated steriliser, but the temperature of boiling water is the same whether you use a milk tin or a steriliser of stainless steel, stamped out in one piece, with electric heating built in, self-acting safety fuses and what have you. It did the job efficiently.

Some of these things may have been mentioned before. But they will bear repetition in view of their apparent triviality—and their real and vital importance. It must be remembered that each and all of them have killed, some of them once, some of them many times. So it is not a bad thing to collect them all together for easy reference. I must confess that some were new to me.

Just for a change a death will now be mentioned which was not strictly due to anæsthesia, but to one of its ancillary techniques, blood transfusion. This life-saving procedure has a small mortality of its own. Mostly due to incompatibility, presumably, for the more deeply this complicated subject is investigated the wider its boundaries appear to be. But this was an unusual, unconventional case, for it was not the patient who died but the donor.[56] A rotary pump was in use to collect and transfuse the blood—the simple and efficient device by which a rotating roller compresses a circle of rubber tubing and drives the blood forward. The simplicity of this idea means that there is nothing to go wrong—in theory. In practice this rotary pump reversed its action and the blood donor died from air embolism. It was found that a safety valve in the pump was out of action, and that reversal could occur if the rotor was in a certain position—a kind of electrical dead centre—and the pump was switched on at the wall plug and not at the pump itself. A condenser was fitted to prevent reversal and a valve was also put into the suction side.

The rotary pump is by no means a new idea. It was developed as soon as flexible watertight tubing was available commercially. The early models were operated by hand and so immune from the particular fault which caused the above accident. It would be difficult to turn a rotary pump the wrong way by hand because the direction of flow is so obvious. The earliest model dates from 1888.[57] It was designed for blood transfusion, but could also be used for aspiration, as a stomach pump or for embalming!

Air embolism more often kills the patient who is being transfused. Keith Simpson[58] described four fatal cases, all of them different. In two of them the apparatus was, somewhat too optimistically, described as foolproof.

In the first instance a large inverted bottle was in use with a positive air pressure inside it produced by a rubber bulb. It was estimated that the contents would last for forty minutes without supervision or attention, so the patient was left for a time. Unfortunately the solution ran more quickly than anticipated; the bottle emptied itself, and as soon as the last drop of liquid disappeared it was followed by a rush of the compressed air which had been pushing the transfusion fluid onwards. In the second case a perished rubber tube was used which did not make an airtight fit on the glass sight feed dropper. It allowed air to enter, sucked in on the injector principle, air which was carried onwards by the flow of fluid. In the third example the ligature was passed through the vein and not round it, and the fourth was due to difficulty in entering the vein. It was only a small air leak in this case, but it was enough—in a very ill patient.

A special device to eliminate air bubbles in transfusion was designed by Leon Longtin of Montreal.[59] It is made by Desberger's Bismol Laboratories, Montreal, under the name of 'Trapair'. A glass trap is inserted in the transfusion tubing by means of two hollow glass legs at the bottom. The top of the trap is closed by a rubber diaphragm. The trap is, of course, partly filled by the transfused liquid, but any air bubbles rise to the top of it and can be drawn off by a syringe needle inserted through the rubber cap. Any other drug can also be injected in this manner.

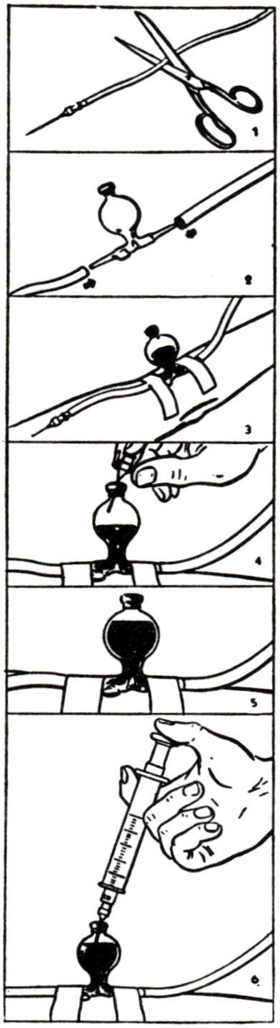

FIG. 5

FIG. 5

Anesthesiology. Leon Longtin, Montreal. Vol. I. 309. 1945. The "Trapair" safety trap for air bubbles in transfusion. The tube is cut, the trap inserted and fixed with plaster. Any air bubbles rise to the top and can be drawn off through the rubber diaphragm. Any drug can also be injected here.

At the risk of repetition there are three other details connected with chloroform anæsthesia not already mentioned in this essay. They are small points which can kill, and have killed, just as surely as the small point of a rapier. The first is, of course, the deadly effect of fear plus light chloroform anæsthesia. Hannah Greener, for example. She had been fretting all the day before "crying continually and wishing she were dead rather than submit to it." These were Dr. Meggison's own words.[60] There was Dr. Roberts' dental case in Edinburgh—the one to which James Y. Simpson was called in a vain attempt to revive her. She had had chloroform five times before without incident. But this time she had heard of a recent death from chloroform in a dental case, and she was very alarmed. How right she was, for she died like a shot rabbit before she was under.

The second is the danger of giving chloroform after an injection of adrenalin. This is really much the same thing as the last, except that in the first case the adrenalin is endogenous, produced by the body itself in a state of fear; in the second it is exogenous, prepared in the laboratory and injected. The effect is the same; the result is the same.

The third detail is the use of chloroform causing delayed chloroform poisoning. It is no use trying to avoid this risk by using small doses, for it has happened (in an adult, mind you, not a child) after as little as four drachms.[61] This was a fatal case, as is usual in this condition.

Intestinal obstruction is well known to be extremely dangerous. From the anæsthetic point of view, in addition to the poor condition of the patient, there is the risk of the lungs being flooded with gastro-intestinal contents. It is not enough to wash out the stomach beforehand and rely on that. Even if the stomach is empty at the end of the wash-out it does not remain so. It is promptly refilled by reverse peristalsis. But this is not a text-book. I must not try to tell you how to do things. The object of this essay is to tell you how not to do them.

Suffice it to say, historically, that one attempt to solve this problem was the use of spinal anæsthesia. It was hoped that retention of consciousness would be a sufficient safeguard. A. Wilfrid Adams tried this method.[62] Analgesia up to the level of the 6th dorsal was induced. But it was of no avail. The patient drowned in his own vomit. No doubt the paralysis of the abdominal muscles and the lower intercostals rendered the patient powerless to get rid of it.

Another form of drowning takes place when a lung abscess floods the sound lung. Here I must mention some personal experiences. Before I retired from anæsthesia I had seen three cases of lung abscess which came to operation. The first one was anæsthetised with cyclopropane, as being a suitable method for general lung surgery, which was then more or less in its infancy. The date must have been later than 1933 (the date of introduction of cyclopropane), but it was not much later. I began to use this gas early, because I had seen the first public demonstration of its use at Madison, Wisconsin, and brought two cylinders of it back with me to England. The dangers of a lung abscess were not fully realised at the time, and unfortunately I took no special precautions. That patient died on the table, his sound lung flooded by the contents of the abscess.

The next case of lung abscess I saw, with the same surgeon, was done under local anæsthesia, to avoid this danger. *But the same thing happened.* Even the presence of a cough reflex and consciousness is of no avail when abscess contents are tilted straight from one main bronchus into the other. They are too far down for any cough to dispose of them with safety.

My third lung abscess was in a prison camp in Eastern Germany. We had quite a nice operating theatre, a reasonable assortment of ordinary instruments, very sketchy anæsthetic equipment—and no frills whatever. We had no such things as bronchoscopes or bronchus blockers. Even the one laryngoscope available had no battery. Our operating table was a light portable model, with a gaspipe frame and a tin top, probably intended for field ambulance use. When this formidable operation was scheduled to be done under these conditions I retired into a corner to think things out. . . . Time to think is the one thing which the prisoner-of-war—or any other prisoner for that matter—possesses in abundance.

My thoughts fell into three groups. First, the sound lung must be protected, as witness my two other cases. Secondly, it must be done by positioning the patient, as we had no other method. Thirdly, the moment of danger is when the cavity is incised. Until then, unless the cavity has a very large opening, nothing will escape from it in any position until the vacuum is broken by an incision.

The position question was solved in this way. Put your left hand flat on the table in front of you, palm downwards. Bend the thumb, ring and little fingers into the palm. They are not wanted for this demonstration. You now have the back of the hand, and the first and middle fingers in full extension. Separate the two fingers as widely as possible. The back of the hand represents the trachea and the V of the fingers the two bronchi. Now dorsiflex the wrist slightly to represent the head-down position. In this posture, which represents the patient lying either on his back or on his face, it will be seen that quite a small angle of tilt is enough to safeguard the lungs. Any fluid coming down either finger will run down the back of the hand if it is tilted quite a small amount.

But now turn the patient on his side, by turning your hand into the midway position between pronation and supination. Separate the fingers as widely as possible, to represent the angle of the diverging bronchi. It will be obvious that anything coming down the top finger will run into the lower finger unless the whole forearm is tilted sufficiently to have *both* bronchi on a down slope. This requires an angle of tilt far steeper than the Trendelenburg position—an angle of at least 45°.

So I consulted with the surgeon and explained all these points tactfully, and told him of my previous experience with lung abscesses. He agreed that the matter was very important, and we held a rehearsal in the operating theatre. Our gaspipe table, though adequate for ordinary purposes, had no fancy positions or adjustments, so we had to obtain our steep slope by mounting the bottom legs on a packing case. Then we found that two orderlies were required to hold the patient's feet to prevent him cascading on to the floor, and to prevent the whole table tipping over. Large valise straps were also used to help. Forty-five degrees is a lot steeper than the steepest gradient on a very severe hill.

Time to think and time to rehearse were privileges which I had never had in peace-time anæsthesia. But they made for safety and paid handsome dividends. The operation went perfectly smoothly, with no difficulty from the unusual position; the anæsthesia was simplicity itself—ether on an open mask. As predicted, nothing happened until the cavity was opened and the vacuum broken. Then came a flood of pus, but not into the other lung. It flowed along the trachea into the nasopharynx and out of the nostrils. A hand operated, home-made suction device cleaned out the nasopharynx, and the patient, a Spaniard in the French Foreign Legion, did very well.

There are no references to these three cases. They have not been published before.

Another personal case may be included here. Death due to a nasal (thin walled) Magill's tube being inserted through the mouth. The lack of protection which is normally given by the nasal walls, together with the more acute bend, led to kinking of the tube and strangulation of the patient.

This case was the last anæsthetic I gave in civil life before I was called up for the army. It was an intracranial tumour, to be done by a general surgeon because the neurosurgeon had been called up. It was rather out of our province, so the surgeon, very rightly, spent a considerable time in the theatre during the morning seeing that everything was properly arranged and just as he wanted it, with the exception, of course, of unimportant details like the anæsthetic. Would that I could have done the same, but that was impossible, owing to the pressure of general practice work, which had to be done. The crazy insistence on cheap anæsthesia was such that I could not make a living out of anæsthetics after twenty years' work, in a town of half a million inhabitants, with about another million within a radius of fifteen miles. I did the best I could in the time available and took a blood pressure apparatus with me and fixed it on the arm. I then intubated—with the wrong tube. When the patient was turned over the blood pressure apparatus was found to be on the wrong arm and quite inaccessible. Remember that everything was done in a frantic hurry, and that I was not used to these cases. I did not even know where the tumour was or what operating position was to be used. Respiratory exchange was unsatisfactory, but by this time the patient had vanished from sight under sterile towels and the operation had begun. Short of stopping the operation altogether and wrecking the whole aseptic set-up nothing could be done about it, so I hoped for the best. This was very unwise, with not even the sphygmomanometer as a control. The kink in the tube was severe and the patient died on the table.

Five years later, after army service had taught me the value of unhurried, thoughtful, leisurely work and the peace of mind ensured by examination of the patients before and after operation, I gave up anæsthesia on my return to England. This case was one of the main reasons. I knew that a full time National Health Service was to be brought in and that conditions would change for the better—but when? Three years later, as a matter of fact. In the meantime I had to choose between general practice and my anæsthetic work. I would no longer even consider doing both and risking further unnecessary deaths, merely by hurried work. But, if I could not make a living out of anæsthesia before the war, after twenty years' continuous work at it, what chance had I now after five years' absence, when new anæsthetists were well established with all the surgeons for whom I used to work? As I have a sneaking prejudice in favour of three meals a day I did the only thing possible and chose general practice. But enough of that. I have now retired from general practice as well, financial considerations have receded into the background of the years, and I am as busy as I ever was in collecting material for, and writing, these essays. I can imagine no greater contentment.

I feel that the occasional insertion of disasters of my own, although I am not proud of them, gives me a certain *locus standi* as a compiler of other people's mistakes. It is certainly an inducement to humility and a wholesome corrective of vanity.

There is one more condition, not very well known, which can cause death during anæsthesia, and that is impaction of the epiglottis into or on to the larynx. F. J. Palmer of Assam[63] reported three cases of sudden respiratory obstruction from this cause. The epiglottis was hooked up and the obstruction freed. In one case this was not possible and he temporarily pushed it down into the glottis until the air could get past it, and then hooked it up. G. H. Caiger says:[64]

"... I had been present at a case of death from respiratory failure ... a few days later I was looking on at an operation on a tonsillar growth (diathermy). Soon after the gag had been placed in position respiration ceased. ... I suggested a digital examination. I found the epiglottis impacted in the larynx, and on this occasion, on being picked up, it flew out with an audible click (this is the only time I have heard it 'click' out). It was audible to those close to the patient's head."

He goes on to say that he had now seen 8 cases, with 4 different anæsthetists, both with ether and chloroform. "In my opinion this type of respiratory failure is more common than is generally recognised, and is probably responsible for a considerable proportion of deaths under anæsthesia."

H. M. Wharry[65] had seen 3 cases of complete and many cases of partial obstruction due to it. He wrote a long article about it in 1927.[66] F. C. Eve saw it, not during anæsthesia but in electrocution.[67] No flow of air could be detected on artificial respiration. Intubation failed. At the post-mortem the epiglottis was sealed down tightly on to the glottis—it had to be lifted with a knife. He remarks that cases have been reported during anæsthesia, and suggests that it may be the cause of some blast deaths from explosions. The danger is greatest when the lungs are empty. The lethal vacuum could be broken by a trocar or large needle in the trachea.

I leave to your consideration, then, thirty-seven baroque methods of killing patients. Until I began to collect them I didn't know there were as many as that; did you?

* * * * * *

April, 1960.—Here is a stop-press item in the daily paper. It comes well outside my hundred year period, so I have not changed the number in the title of this essay. But I had to mention it as yet another unusual cause of death. A patient was electrocuted by a cardiac monitor machine.

References

[1] *Lancet* (1873), May 24. 749.
[2] *Lancet* (1873), June 14. 846.
[3] K. Wilson (1899), *Lancet*, June 24. 1727.
[4] *Lancet* (1889), July 27. 184.
[5] *Lancet* (1894), May 26. 1354.
[6] John T. Bouchier-Hayes (1906). *Brit. med. J.*, Nov. 10. 1343.
[7] F. E. Junker (1867). *Med. Times Gaz.*, Nov. 30. 590.
[8] Rickard W. Lloyd (1917). *Lancet*, July 21. 97.
[9] Joseph Mills (1878). *Lancet*, Dec. 14. 839.
[10] Krohne & Sesemann (1883). *Brit. med. J.*, Apr. 28. 821.
[11] Dudley Buxton (1884). *Lancet*, Oct. 4. 595.
[12] Krohne & Sesemann (1891). *Brit. med. J.*, June 27. 1389.
[13] Frederic Hewitt (1892). *Lancet*, Apr. 30. 966.
[14] Carter Braine (1892). *Brit. med. J.*, June 25. 1364.
[15] W. J. Foster (1927). *Brit. med. J.*, Feb. 5. 261.
[16] *Lancet* (1928), Dec. 29. 1352.
[17] C. F. Hadfield (1919). *Brit. med. J.*, Mar. 22. 359.
[18] *Brit. med. J.* (1931), May 23. 915.
[19] Thomas Nunneley (1849). *Trans. Prov. med. surg. Assoc.* XVI.
[20] J. Mason Warren (1868). *History of Anaesthesia from an American point of View.*
[21] H. W. Featherstone (1931). *Proc. R. Soc. Med.* Vol. 25, 119.
[22] R. Ironside (1935). *Proc. R. Soc. Med.* Vol. 28, 1127.
[23] G. Ramsey Phillips (1931). *Proc. R. Soc. Med.* Vol. 25, 119.
[24] *Brit. med. J.* (1925), Oct. 17. 713.
[25] *Brit. med. J.* (1926), Jan. 30. 207.
[26] Bernard D. Bolas (1925). *Brit. med. J.*, Nov. 28. 1035.
[27] J. N. Loring (1925). *Brit. med. J.*, Dec. 26. 1246.
[28] B. B. Lennon and E. A. Rovenstine (1939). *Curr. Res. Anesth.* 18, 218.
[29] H. D. Gillies, T. Pomfret Kilner and A. H. McIndoe (1940). *Brit. med. J.*, Jan. 13. 69.
[30] Geoffrey Kaye (1935). *Brit. med. J.*, Oct. 5. 618.
[31] *Brit. med. J.* (1940), Mar. 16. 470.
[32] *Brit. med. J.* (1944), Oct. 28. 582.
[33] *Brit. med. J.* (1945), Mar. 17. 381.
[34] *Lancet* (1945), Sept. 1. 278.
[35] J. S. Lundy (1942). *Clinical Anesthesia.* Philadelphia: Saunders.
[36] American Medical Association (1954). *Fundamentals of Anesthesia.* Philadelphia: Saunders.
[37] F. R. Brown (1940). *Brit. med. J.*, Oct. 12. 503.
[38] C. J. Massey Dawkins (1940). *Brit. med. J.*, Oct. 19. 587.
[39] C. Langton Hewer and C. F. Hadfield (1941). *Brit. med. J.*, June 21. 924.
[40] J. H. Humphrey and Margaret McClelland (1944). *Brit. med. J.*, Mar. 4. 315.
[41] S. Carden (1944). *Brit. med. J.*, Mar. 4.
[42] *Brit. med. J.* (1944), Mar. 25. 434.
[43] *Lancet* (1937), Apr. 24. 1006.
[44] *Lancet* (1939), Oct. 28. 944.
[45] *Lancet* (1942), Aug. 22. 221.
[46] *Lancet* (1942), Sept. 19. 340.

[47] Geoffrey Organe (1942). *Lancet*, July 11. 33.
[48] *Lancet* (1942), Aug. 1. 134.
[49] *Lancet* (1936), May 14. 623.
[50] *Lancet* (1941), Feb. 22. 242.
[51] C. L. Hewer and L. P. Garrod (1942). *Lancet*, Feb. 28. 275.
[52] *Lancet* (1945), Jan. 27. 115.
[53] *Lancet* (1945), Mar. 3. 286.
[54] *Lancet* (1945), Mar. 3, 287.
[55] *Lancet* (1945), Mar. 17. 352.
[56] *Brit. med. J.* (1941), Aug. 30. 311.
[57] *Brit, med. J.* (1888), Sept. 29. 722.
[58] Keith Simpson (1942). *Lancet*, June 13. 697.
[59] Leon Longtin (1945). *Anesthesiology*. Vol. 6, p. 309.
[60] Dr. Meggison (1848). *Med. Tms.*, Feb. 5. 317.
[61] T. F. Todd (1934). *Lancet*, Sept. 15. 597.
[62] A. Wilfrid Adams (1931). *Brit. med. J.*, May 9. 785.
[63] F. J. Palmer (1924). *Brit. med. J.*, Feb. 23. 353.
[64] G. H. Caiger (1927). *Brit. med. J.*, Aug. 6. 238.
[65] H. M. Wharry (1942). *Brit. med. J.*, Sept. 19. 344.
[66] H. M. Wharry (1927). *Brit. med. J.*, May 21. 914.
[67] F. C. Eve (1943). *Lancet*, June 26. 799.

CHAPTER 2

ANÆSTHETIC DEATHS IN THE FIRST HUNDRED YEARS

OCCASIONALLY, in searching through the literature, one finds anæsthetists or surgeons quoting the numbers of anæsthetic deaths for a few years in order to prove some particular point or to back up some argument; but nowhere did I discover any attempt to take the large view. Nobody ever endeavoured to find out the total number of deaths over a long period. So far as I know this has never been done.

John Snow did make an attempt to do it at the beginning, and in fact, collected a list of fifty deaths in the first ten years. No doubt he would have continued to keep the score if he had lived longer. But he died in 1858, and nobody else bothered about it. The deaths in Snow's list were distributed as follows; 25 from England and Wales, 6 from Scotland and 19 from the rest of the world. These figures are evidently incomplete, as is shown by their lack of balance. It is inconceivable that the whole of the rest of the world should produce a lesser number of deaths than England and Wales alone; the obvious explanation is that foreign deaths were less likely to be reported in the English journals than those which occurred nearer home.

Here again, by the way, is another opportunity to test the truth of the legend that chloroform was perfectly safe when given in Scotland. The figures are too small to be really reliable, but, such as they are they are worth examining. The population of England and Wales at that time was 6·26 times as large as that of Scotland;[1] if the death rates were equal England should have had 37 deaths instead of 25. Or, alternatively, if the English rate is taken as the standard, Scotland should have had 4 deaths only instead of 6.

After Snow's death there were few other attempts to cope with an ever-increasing problem. Henry M. Lyman's[2] was perhaps the best. Well over fifty pages of his book are occupied by case reports of 393 chloroform deaths collected from all sources. Fifteen died at the beginning of the inhalation, and 99 before complete insensibility. Seventy died during and 35 after the operation. Inhalers were used in 46 cases, towel or lint in 139. Six of the patients were in labour. Lyman reports a further

17 deaths from mixtures or sequences containing chloroform, 27 deaths from ether and 8 from nitrous oxide. One of these was due to the inhalation of a loose cork used as a dental prop, which was hardly the fault of the nitrous oxide, though it was the fault of the anæsthetist.

The indefatigable Dr. Lyman also quotes several large series of cases collected by others:

Andrews of Chicago collected—

Chloroform	117,078 with	43 deaths or 1 in	2,723.
Ether	92,815 with	4 deaths or 1 in	23,204.
Mixtures	11,176 with	2 deaths or 1 in	5,588.
Bichloride of methylene	7,000 with	1 death or 1 in	7,000.

Coles of Virginia reported—

Chloroform	152,620 with	53 deaths or 1 in	2,873.
Methylene bichloride	10,000 with	2 deaths or 1 in	5,000.

B. W. Richardson—

Chloroform	35,165 with	11 deaths or 1 in	3,196.

Billroth of Vienna claimed—

Chloroform	12,500 with	1 death,

but this estimate appears to be somewhat optimistic, because there are no less than four deaths reported in Billroth's practice before this date.[3]

Many other large series reported by Lyman were apparently mere estimates, as they all ended in a neat row of noughts. I always look with grave suspicion on statistics in even thousands, as they are invariably pure guesswork.

The largest collected series of cases which I found was that of Julliard[4]:—

Chloroform	524,507 with	161 deaths or 1 in	3,258.
Ether	314,738 with	21 deaths or 1 in	14,987.

Chloroform invariably heads the list with round about one death in every three thousand, but the whole position as regards the total deaths over the whole period seemed to be so vague and nebulous that I thought something ought to be done about it.

The vast catalogue of the Cambridge University Library did not mention the Registrar General's reports, so I enquired about them and was referred to the Official Publications Department, who very soon told me where the reports were kept. So I began to work my way through them, which took about three days. The more recent ones were easy, in that there was a special section devoted to anæsthetics, but they were slow and tedious to abstract because the tables of deaths were so long and detailed. In the 1949 report for example, no less than 141 different methods, mixtures and sequences are listed to account for the 704 deaths, covering three pages of small print. This was a vast change from the stark simplicity of the early reports, which listed chloroform only, and their immediate successors which added nitrous oxide in 1873 and ether in 1875 as a concession to anæsthetic progress. But to offset their simplicity the figures in the early reports were much more difficult to find, for they were not mentioned in the index or the table of contents. They were also apt to disappear and to turn up again, after a long search, under a different heading. At one time they were classified under Deaths from Accident and Violence, subsection Asphyxia, together with curious causes of death such as Cat on Face (which occurred more than once), gas ovens, judicial executions, and so on. Then all would be plain sailing for twenty years or so until the Registrar General changed his mind and put them somewhere else.

I eventually managed to track down the required figures as far back as 1868, with two volumes missing from the series (which I later obtained from the Leeds University Library). Then I lost the trail completely and finally. So the earlier years of the chart had to be filled up, partly from John Snow's figures for the first ten years, then by case reports from the *Lancet* and some figures given by the *British Medical Journal.* These sources were not necessarily complete and almost certainly omitted an unknown number of cases, but it was the best I could do.

I wrote to the Registrar General later and he confirmed the fact that the figures before 1868 did not exist in any records at his office. He added that figures from any sources for the period in question would probably be unreliable. That, of course, I knew already.

Having searched through all these volumes for the mortality in England and Wales, I turned wearily to the annual reports for Scotland —and failed to find the required data at all. By this time I felt that I had been immersed in masses of figures for all eternity, so I gave up the search. The figures must be there somewhere, I suppose, for Glaister[5] gives the total for Scotland as 103 in 1927. He gave the score for England and Wales for the same year as 596, which agrees exactly with my own figures extracted from the annual reports.

If one works out these two totals as a proportion of the population at the nearest Census the deaths in Scotland were 1 in 47,000 compared with 1 in 67,000 for England and Wales. Or if we give the benefit of the doubt to Scotland and assume that the Scottish mortality rate was the same as the English all the time, in spite of the above figures, we must then add 4,212 deaths to the 24,378 which occurred in England and Wales, making a grand total of 28,590 for Great Britain, excluding Ireland. This does not sound unreasonable for the hundred years, when one considers that the two Glaisters[6] did 444 post-mortems on anæsthetic deaths in the thirty years 1899-1929 in the district of Glasgow and the West of Scotland alone. This was before the really big increase in the number of operations, for the most part; only the last seven years of the thirty come into this period.

It must be remembered that this Scottish total is only an estimate, but it is based on some sort of evidence and is probably somewhere near the truth. If I ever do trace the figures for Scotland I should certainly prefer them to any estimate, however careful.

But it is essential to be fair. At an earlier period, when the figures were smaller, F. J. Waldo, Coroner for the City of London and Southwark,[7] gave some figures for Scotland which show that country in a rather more favourable light. He says that the deaths for England and Wales for 1905 were 155, which again is correct according to my chart. The Scottish deaths for the same year were 18. At the 1911 Census the population of England and Wales was 7·57 times that of Scotland. This means that Scotland would have had 20 deaths instead of 18 if the rate had been the same as in England; or that the English deaths would have been 136 instead of 155 if they had been at the same rate as the Scottish deaths. So Scotland is in the lead during this particular year.

When I was searching the journals and card-indexing every reference to anæsthesia, I made one exception to this rule. I did not devote a separate card to every anæsthetic death reported, because many of the reports were so defective in detail that they merely recorded a death; and I thought that I could always get a more accurate record of the mere numbers from the Registrar's reports.

But in some cases there were special features of interest which led me to make out a card for them. All deaths from anæsthesia are tragic, with the possible exception of those which occur during an attempt to save a patient from inevitable death; deaths during trivial operations are particularly distressing, because they are such a wanton and unnecessary waste. There were two cases which excelled all others in this respect; both of them occurred in the United States. In 1872 Dr. Asa Wheat of Canaan gave his wife chloroform for dental extractions. The dentist, his brother, had taken out three teeth when she died.[8] Eleven years later the same tragedy happened to an unfortunate doctor in Philadelphia. After the removal of one tooth the wife-patient was found to be dead.[9]

In 1899 there was a very black week in which no fewer than nine deaths under chloroform were reported in one issue of the *Lancet*.[10] Two of them happened in Liverpool, four in various London hospitals, two in military hospitals and one at Dudley.

Joseph Thomas Clover, one of the first professional anæsthetists, was born on February 28th, 1825. He went to University College Hospital in 1844 and was present at Liston's first operation under ether.[11] He became Resident Medical Officer at the hospital in 1848 and was later chloroformist to it, and also to the Westminster and the Dental Hospital. He stated in 1871[12] that he had given chloroform more than 7000 times, in addition to other anæsthetics in another 4000 cases.

"I have never drawn out the tongue, and never lost a patient from any anæsthetic. Raising the chin is sufficient. It is my habit . . . to watch the pulse as well as the breathing, and I am therefore better able to speak of the effect of chloroform upon the heart than those who disregard the pulse."

He goes on to describe a case in which the pulse gave him the first warning of danger. Sixteen months later his clean record was still unbroken.[13] Clover's method then was in direct opposition to that of Syme and Lawrie, and was equally successful. He had, however, seen a chloroform death in 1853.[14] Chloroform was given by a student in the hospital to a woman of 28 for the application of nitric acid to sloughing ulcers of the labia. The student sent for Clover, then the R.M.O., when the death occurred. Clover stated that chloroform had been given 1600 times in the hospital in the last four years with but one fatal case—presumably this one.

In 1874, however, Clover had a chloroform death himself. (*Brit. med. J.*, 1874, June 20. 817.)

A case of fatal syncope during the administration of chloroform. Mr. J. T. Clover sends us the following note.

In the following notes two modes of giving chloroform are alluded to. The first is what is known as "Clover's chloroform apparatus," consisting of a bag (in this instance charged with a mixture of thirty-two minims of chloroform, four of ether, and one thousand cubic inches of air—[=16,387 cc.]) from which bag the patient inhales by means of a tube and valved face-piece. The second is called "the blowing apparatus", (Junker's apparatus was first described in the *Medical Times and Gazette*, 1867, Nov. 30, 590) and consists of a bellows moved by the foot, which drives air through a vessel containing chloroform, and forwards by means of a tube held in, or near, the patient's mouth or nose. A stopcock regulates or stops the current. It is intended only for operations in which the first instrument cannot be applied.

On June 13th, 1874, Mr. John Marshall was about to remove some adenoid growths from the posterior nares of a gentleman. It was likely to be a tedious operation, and, for its effective performance, the patient must be kept quiet as well as insensible. The patient was seated on a chair, much reclining backwards. A piece of vulcanite, with string attached to it, was put between his teeth, and he commenced inhaling from the bag apparatus. He inhaled well, but swallowed frequently. At the end of five minutes, he vomited three or four ounces of yellow matter. After the retching ceased, he began talking, but leaned back quietly, and took the anæsthetic for three or four minutes, when Mr. Marshall began to explore the nostril and fauces. This produced some retching, and he became unsteady, so that I found the blowing apparatus I had just applied inconvenient. I put it aside, and a third time used the bag apparatus, until the cornea was insensitive, and the pupils well contracted. His pulse was regular, but a little diminished in force at this time, about fifteen minutes from the commencement of inhaling. I now finally put down the bag inhaler, and the prop having been adjusted, Mr. Marshall again made an examination of the growth, and was beginning to put a ligature through the nostril into the mouth. I was thus delayed using the blowing apparatus a minute or so, and the patient became half conscious, and leaned forward voluntarily; but he was not sick. On renewing the application of chloroformed air by the tube, he drew in so much fresh air along with it that, in order to make the instrument effective, I placed a cambric handkerchief lightly over the face, watching the pulse carefully at the same time. In less than half a minute after this, he seemed about to vomit, and his pulse became weak, but not weaker than is usual when vomiting takes place under chloroform. I removed the handkerchief and chloroform, and was about to hold a basin under his chin whilst his head was raised, but noticing that he was pale and his pupils dilated, we placed him at once recumbent upon the floor. He breathed slowly and with remarkable freedom; and as the respirations became less effective, we assisted them artificially by the Sylvester and Baines's method. The prop remained in its place, and by keeping the mouth open assisted the access of fresh air. There was no difficulty about this getting through the larynx. It passed without an audible noise, and without any check. He moaned three or four times, and once or twice I thought I could feel the pulse, but the pupils never regained their natural size. In about quarter of an hour there seemed to be a little mucus in the air-passages. Ammonia was held near the mouth, cold water dashed on the face, hot cloths applied over the chest, and artificial respiration was kept up for an hour, when it was evidently useless to continue it longer.

Remarks.—No opportunity of examining the heart after death was afforded us. There may have been something besides chloroform to cause death, but I cannot hold the chloroform blameless, and am inclined to think that, when the handkerchief was applied like a veil over the face, the vapour became too strong for an enfeebled heart. Although I have used the blowing apparatus so many times with marked success, and might use it again a thousand times without meeting with the conditions to cause a like result, I shall not use it again until some plan can be devised for making it an impossibility to give a stronger percentage of vapour than experience with the bag inhaler makes me believe to be quite safe. Whether it caused the catastrophe or not, the exchange of the bag apparatus for the blowing instrument was so quickly followed by alarming symptoms, that I cannot help suspecting it yielded the chloroform too freely.

It will occur to many who have used ether as an anæsthetic that this would have been a safer agent. But it should be remembered that there were special reasons here for avoiding irritating the throat, and I had noticed that the very small quantity put into the bag inhaler, caused frequent swallowing.

Ether can indeed be introduced so gradually as to produce very little irritation, by the aid of nitrous oxide. I have already so used it in more than four hundred cases, without any untoward result, and with immense comfort to the patient as compared with the ordinary way of giving ether, but I did not think this a fit case for using a combination which must, as yet, be considered as upon its trial. Perhaps it is fortunate that I did not, for it might have been supposed to have had more to do with causing death than the method adopted, whose use has been established for many years.

In the next case of this sort, I intend to give ether with gas, and then ether with a limited supply of air for at least ten minutes; and if I give any chloroform after this, it should be still more diluted than it was in this unhappy case.

W. A. Parker[15] of Lancaster asked an extremely silly question in 1895. "Why do we almost never have a report of a death under chloroform from Scotland, where practically nothing else is used? I believe that they are not afraid of it and push it rapidly." A little thought might have solved his problem easily. At the Census of 1891 the population of England was 7·45 times as big as that of Scotland. In 1901 it was 7·27 times as big. So it would not be unreasonable to expect Mr. Parker to deduce that Scottish deaths would probably be only about one-seventh the number of those in England. Secondly, there were no inquests in Scotland, which would tend to reduce the number of newspaper reports of Scottish deaths to an even lower level. Thirdly, deaths did occur, and were reported—or some of them.

James Spence, Professor of Surgery at Edinburgh, admitted that "seven or eight cases (*i.e.* deaths) . . . have occurred in the Royal Infirmary in 32 years. . . ."[16] A death took place before the operation began in Mr. Chiene's ward a few weeks later.[17] A young boy died at Glasgow

CHART I

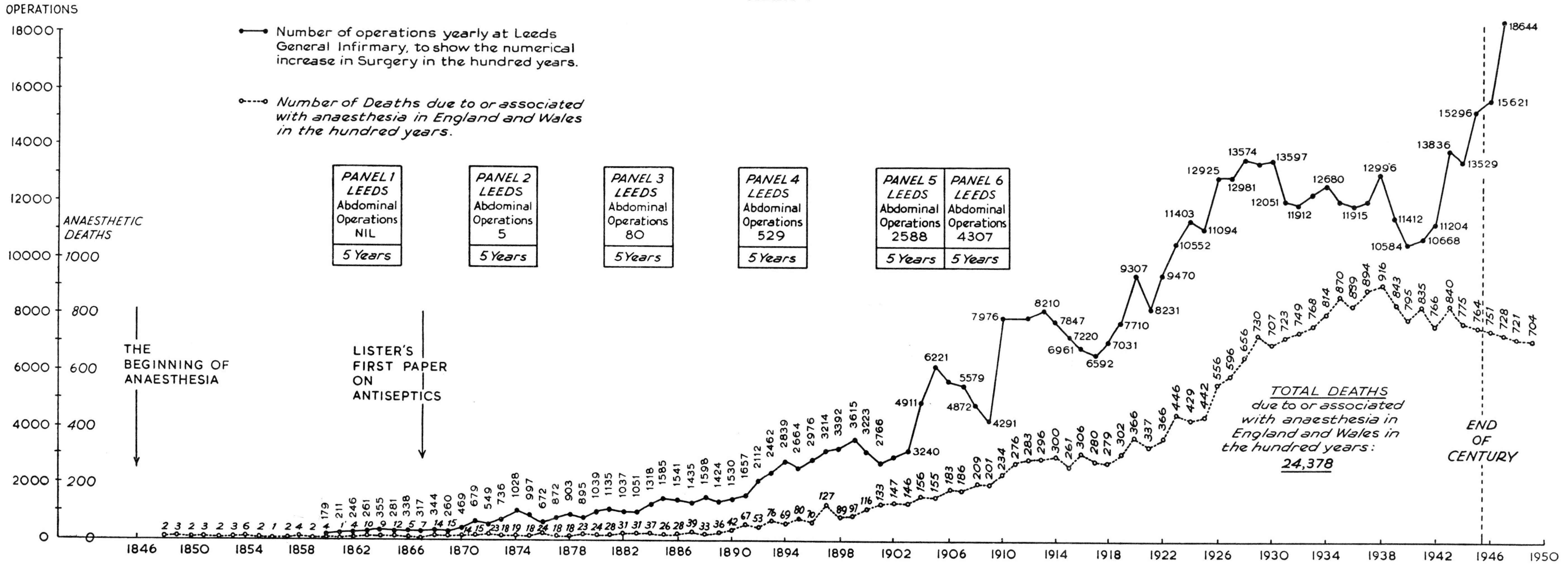

The first 5 panels on the chart were taken from figures given by T. Pridgin Teale, F.R.C.S., Consulting Surgeon to the Leeds General Infirmary in a speech at King's College Hospital. (*Lancet, 1906, Oct. 13. 977*, and *Brit. med. J., 1906, Oct. 6. 828*.) Dr. Stephen Anning, who is writing a history of the Infirmary for its bi-centenary, pointed out to me that panel 1 omits any reference to ovariotomies. During that period (1961-65) 16 of these were performed with 11 deaths, or 68·7 per cent. Why Mr. Teale did not include these I do not know; especially as he and another surgeon were given permission in 1864, according to Dr. Anning, to take private lodgings near the Infirmary in order to perform operations for "ovarian dropsy". This was a common practice at that time. The dirt of an ordinary house was thought to be less dangerous than the pathogenic dirt of a hospital. Perhaps this belief originated from Simpson's work on Hospitalism (See Vol. I of these Essays, p. 130.)

The remainder of the figures on the chart were obtained by me direct from the Annual Reports, whenever possible.

CHART II

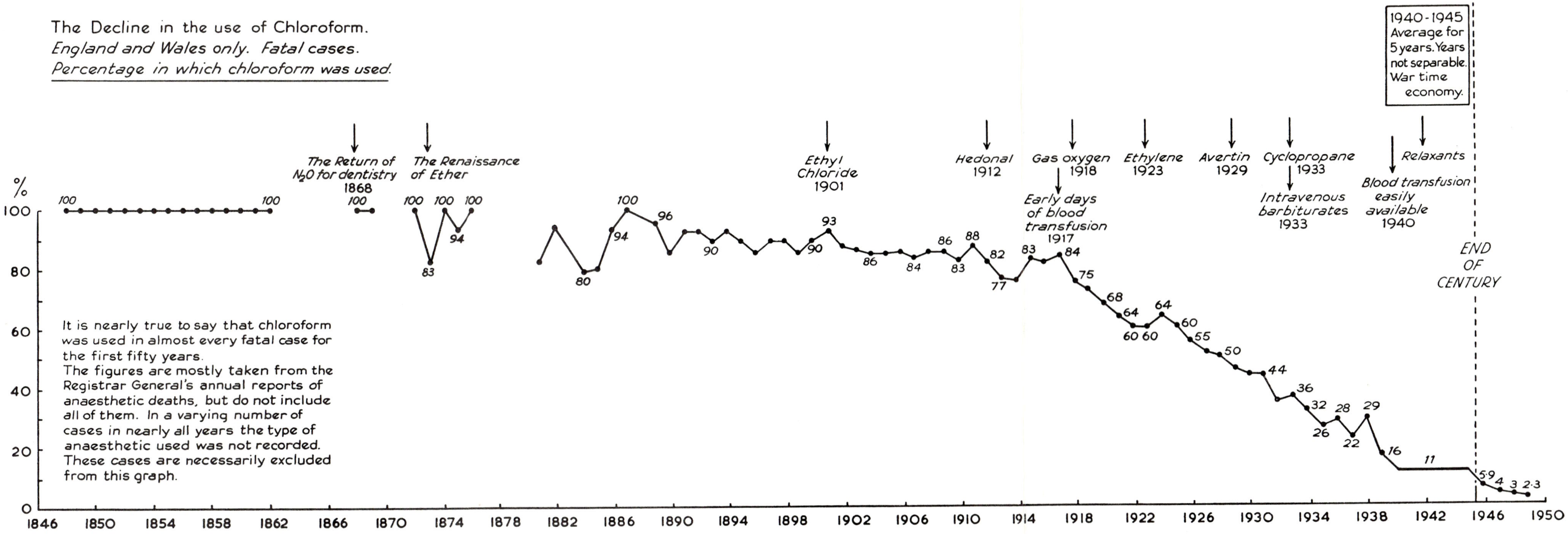

The Decline in the use of Chloroform.
England and Wales only. Fatal cases.
Percentage in which chloroform was used.
The Return of N₂O for dentistry 1868
The Renaissance of Ether
Ethyl Chloride 1901
Hedonal 1912
Gas oxygen 1918
Early days of blood transfusion 1917
Ethylene 1923
Avertin 1929
Cyclopropane 1933
Intravenous barbiturates 1933
Relaxants
Blood transfusion easily available 1940
1940-1945 Average for 5 years. Years not separable. War time economy.
END OF CENTURY
It is nearly true to say that chloroform was used in almost every fatal case for the first fifty years.
The figures are mostly taken from the Registrar General's annual reports of anaesthetic deaths, but do not include all of them. In a varying number of cases in nearly all years the type of anaesthetic used was not recorded. These cases are necessarily excluded from this graph.
%

Royal Infirmary in 1884.[18] A year before this a death took place—the third—at the Glasgow Western Infirmary.[19]

But not all the deaths were reported. Dr. Hughes Bennett said:[20]

" . . . a young and beautiful lady, daughter of a barrister, in perfect health, went to a dentist's house one morning and had a tooth extracted. Five minutes afterwards she was dead. That was only one of many similar cases that had occurred, *but had never been published.*"

It was praiseworthy of Dr. Bennett to bring this case to the light of day, but difficult to understand the stress laid on the beauty of the patient. Surely the lives of those less beautiful are of equal importance?

Deaths happened in other towns, too. A man of 37 died on the first incision at Aberdeen Royal Infirmary.[21] But the catalogue need not be continued. No city was immune.

No country was immune, either. Figures were given[22] for Scandinavia for the period February, 1894, to May, 1895.

Chloroform	11,047 with 5 deaths or 1 in 2,209.
Ether	1,279 with 0 deaths.
C.E. mixtures	2,122 with 0 deaths.
Ethyl bromide	367 with 0 deaths.
Total	14,815.

No age was immune. Frank Shearer[23] reported a death at the age of 17 months.

"Previous to the occurrence of this case I shared the impression . . . that as Mr. Lister puts it . . . young children enjoyed an immunity from danger. In eleven years I found 3 deaths under five out of a total of 70 from chloroform in England."

Mr. Robert Bell of Glasgow was a muddle-headed gentleman[24] who began by compiling a list of inquests in England for the year 1897. According to him there were 26 in private patients and 70 in hospital cases. Of these 96 patients (the Registrar General's figures for this year are 127), 84 had chloroform or mixtures containing it, 7 had ether, 2 nitrous oxide and ether, while 3 had nitrous oxide alone. However accurate or inaccurate Mr. Bell's facts are, his next statement is merely fatuous:

Two deaths from chloroform per year in Snow's days—1848 to 1850—against 96 deaths from anæsthetics in 1897 clearly shows that instead of improving the method of administration, the work of anæsthetics has greatly deteriorated.

He calmly ignores completely the enormous increase in the number of anæsthetics given and the increase in severity of many of the operations, for 1897 was well into the era of abdominal surgery. In other words he compares two entirely different things—pre-Listerian surgery and Listerian surgery.

He then gives a series of very confused statistics. He begins by saying that in the 12 years between 1848 and 1863 there were 86 deaths or 7·1 per year. It is difficult to know from his wording whether he intends to include or exclude one or both of the years mentioned, but in any case his arithmetic is wrong, so there is no profit in following him any further. The period from 1848 to 1863 can be 14, 15 or 16 years according to choice, but in no case can it be 12 years.

Lauder Brunton put forward the theory that irritation of the fifth cranial nerve during light chloroform anæsthesia would produce slowing and finally stoppage of the heart through the vagus.[25] This was intended to explain dental fatalities. But many other minor operations such as removal of the toe-nail had a particularly bad reputation for their liability to stop the heart under (or partially under) chloroform, and by no stretch of the imagination could the vagus, or the fifth nerve, be connected, directly or indirectly, with the toe-nail.

Edward Lawrie, of Hyderabad, said, years later,[26] with reference to another theory from the same source:

> Dr. Brunton . . . considered that there was no danger with chloroform in capital operations like amputations of the leg or arm, but that the special danger with chloroform lay in minor operations like . . . cutting out the toe nail. I well recollect Dr. Bomford saying, when he propounded these views, that if they were correct all that was necessary to make safe the operation of cutting out the toe nail under chloroform would be for the patient first to have his leg off.

In any case, Lawrie attached no importance whatever to the action of the vagus in slowing or stopping the heart, which he considered to be a sort of safety device. One of his most astounding statements was to this effect:[27]

> (Dr. C. Smith's case) affords a striking example of the danger of pulse feeling in chloroform administration. It is clear from Dr. Colvin Smith's account of the case that the heart was refusing to convey any more chloroform to the brain at this time—i.e., while the cyanosis lasted. If the patient had only been left alone, and the safeguard action of the vagus had not been

frustrated by the injection of ether, *the stoppage of the heart would have saved his life.* (My italics).

Lawrie ignored completely the almost worldwide and universal experience of the profession that stoppage of the heart was, in a large proportion of cases, utterly final and irrevocable.

Many of the deaths were quite simply due to incompetent anæsthesia, which allowed the operation to begin when the patient was by no means under. Mr. Crane[28] reported a case in Kent—a man of 49 who was to have some diseased bone removed from his foot. The patient winced on incision, then struggled and sat up in bed!

Robert Kirk brought forward a new theory in 1891.[29] He held that the danger of chloroform lay in interrupting the administration. Once begun, he said, go on regardless of the pulse or anything else until full anæsthesia has been attained. There were two important points[30]—the percentage of vapour used and the length of time of inhalation. He agreed with Dr. Snow that anything above 5 per cent. was dangerous. But there are two zones below this—(1) varying from 1½ per cent. to 3½ per cent. which is safe *provided that* the inhalation is carried to deep anæsthesia, but liable to give a dangerous reaction if stopped at the superficial stage, and (2) a still weaker percentage which may be free from any danger of reaction.

In practice this theory became one of large doses. Dr. Freeland Fergus[31] stated that this Dr. Robert Kirk of Partick had frequently given anæsthetics for him during the last year. In no case had there been any trouble. But he gives no indication whether this applies to a dozen cases or a thousand. Dr. Kirk was in the habit of giving huge doses. A child of ten years old had two ounces of chloroform for the enucleation of an eye.

Specialist anæsthetists, then as now, were not immune from fatal cases. Mr. Potter, assistant apothecary to St. George's Hospital, had his first death from chloroform in 1,400 cases in 1854.[32] The patient was very nervous and apprehensive. She died in one and a half minutes after inhaling about 20 minims of chloroform. Mr. Edwards, chloroformist to St. Mary's Hospital, had his first death in ten years in 1861. His experience covered over 4,000 cases.[33]

Sir Bernard Spilsbury, the pathologist, reported in 1923[34] that he had examined 278 cases of death under anæsthesia, not including delayed chloroform poisoning. Of these, 58 were associated with status lymphaticus; 192 of them (69 per cent.) had had chloroform or mixtures, 48 had ether, 10 stovaine, and 17 nitrous oxide.

The Glaisters, father and son, only saw 7 deaths which they attributed to status lymphaticus in their series of 444 post-mortems on Scottish victims of anæsthesia.[35]

The charts of anæsthetic deaths

The graphs show several interesting features. The decline in the use of chloroform is very clearly indicated. While it is nearly true to say that chloroform was almost exclusively used until 1917 (or at any rate, in never less than three-quarters of the fatal cases) it fell rapidly out of favour after this date, which was about the time Boyle introduced his gas-oxygen apparatus.

Although the percentage of fatal cases in which chloroform was used decreased rapidly, the actual number of deaths was rising with such speed during the fourth quarter of the century, that in actual fact the largest number of chloroform deaths ever recorded in one year—278—occurred in 1933, although this only rated a percentage of 36.

The figures given on the chloroform chart are taken from the annual anæsthetic deaths, but do not include all of them. In a varying number of cases in almost all years the type of anæsthesia used was not recorded, and these had to be deducted before calculating the percentages.

The re-introduction of nitrous oxide in 1868, mainly for dentistry, by T. W. Evans of Paris, and the re-introduction of ether in 1873 by Joy Jeffries of Boston, did not have any appreciable effect on the curve of deaths. The numbers were small at that date, in any case.

Abdominal surgery was practically unknown before 1870, except for a few pioneer belly-rippers, as the ovariotomists were contemptuously called. It was even rare in the early 1880's, though some of the first ovariotomists had done large numbers of cases by this time. The first heroic surgeon to perform a successful ovariotomy was Ephraim McDowell of Kentucky,[36] who was born on November 11th, 1771. On December 13th, 1809, Mrs. Crawford rode sixty miles to Danville to see him. She had an ovarian cyst, which he removed in twenty-five minutes through a nine-inch incision. It weighed 22½ lb., quite a small one by the standards of those days. It was, of course, long before Listerism and long before anæsthesia. The ordeal for the patient was appalling, the risk enormous, and, what was not calculated to comfort the surgeon or steady his nerves, there was a crowd waiting outside to lynch him if the patient died. The patient did not die—not until thirty-three years later, at the age of seventy-eight. Altogether the intrepid McDowell did eight cases, with one death.

Charles Clay, of Manchester, removed his first ovarian cyst on September 27th, 1842, and eventually did 395 cases with 101 deaths. Baker Brown, the fearless man who operated upon his own sister, did 9 operations with 7 deaths, and gave it up for a while. Spencer Wells attempted his first ovarian operation in December, 1857, but could not complete it. His first completed operation was in February, 1858. By 1862[37] he had done 50 cases with 17 deaths (34 per cent.). On Friday, June 11th, 1880, he did his 1,000th case, with 232 deaths (23·2 per cent.), and he was one of the more successful operators. Only a few men were rash enough—or brave enough—to do this work with its heavy mortality, although, in hard, cold fact, it was no greater than the ordinary mortality of amputations at that time.

They had this much justification—that ovarian cysts, left alone or treated medically, grew to sizes which are unknown today. Even when non-malignant they were always fatal, because their mere size and weight overwhelmed the patient and crushed her to death. The largest removed by Spencer Wells weighed 125 lbs., and this by no means held the record. Elizabeth Reifsnyder[38] removed one of 169 lb. (12 st. 1 lb., or just over $1\frac{1}{2}$ cwt.). The patient from which it was removed weighed 77 lb. ($5\frac{1}{2}$ st.) or considerably less than half the weight of her tumour.

Lawson Tait of Birmingham was one of Spencer Well's most active rivals. He had completed 1,000 abdominal sections by 1885,[39] and claimed to have had only 93 deaths or 9·3 per cent. A slight doubt was cast upon his statistical accuracy by J. Knowsley Thornton, who commented:[40]

Up to August 5th, 1882, Mr. Tait had performed 226 ovariotomies, with 27 deaths. Up to Dec. 11th, 1882, he claims 312 ovariotomies with only 26 deaths. It follows that between Aug. 5th and Dec. 11th one patient must have come to life again. . . .

A criticism which, if it was well founded, must have been somewhat difficult to answer.

Thomas Keith, of Edinburgh, another ovariotomist, compared his statistics before and after the Listerian revolution.[41] Without antiseptics his results over 14 years gave a mortality of 1 in 7 (14·28 per cent.). Since using the carbolic spray he had only 2 deaths in 49 cases, or 4 per cent.

Statistics are always difficult to compare. I found this when I was wading through a hundred years of annual reports. And I was fortunate in that I had to go no further back than the middle of the nineteenth century. The comparability of earlier statistics, taken from the Bill of Mortality for 1629,[42] say, would indeed be difficult, with entries like Tissicke and Rising of the Lights.

Lister's first paper on antiseptic surgery was published in 1867, and it was not for some years that surgeons, even the most progressive, had sufficient confidence in it or knowledge of it to encroach on hitherto forbidden territory. The rise of abdominal surgery is indicated in the numbered panels on the main chart. These show the number of abdominal operations at various dates in the Leeds General Infirmary—a large teaching hospital in a town of half a million inhabitants (now), surrounded by a very thickly populated area.

Panel 1.	5 years	1861-65	..	nil.
Panel 2.	,,	1871-75	..	5
Panel 3.	,,	1881-85	..	80
Panel 4.	,,	1891-95	..	529
Panel 5.	,,	1901-05	..	2,588
Panel 6.	,,	1906-10	..	4,307

Even this does not represent the true increase in the volume of surgery. The total operations at this hospital in the year 1935 were 12,046, but at about this time the old poor law institutions were being converted into general hospitals. St. James's Hospital, Leeds, was one of these, and it rapidly accumulated a large operating list. By 1955 9,047 operations were performed here, in addition to those of the main teaching hospital.

There is also the increase in severity and duration of operations to be considered. In the same year—1935—at the Leeds Infirmary there were 29 cerebral operations with 9 deaths, and 43 thoracic operations with 4 deaths. There is no reason to think that this one town is any different from other towns of the same size.

Before 1911 any death certificates mentioning anæsthesia, which also mentioned strangulated hernia or cancer, were allocated, not to anæsthesia, but to the surgical condition. This practice was altered in 1911, with the result that the previous figures were really an underestimate and too small. Even the Registrar General quailed at the impossible task of tracing the old death certificates among the millions which had been filed away under what was now an erroneous classification. All he could do was to give figures for the years *after* 1910 and state by how much the numbers should be reduced to render them comparable to the old ones. This would merely involve a count of the certificates as they came in, which mentioned anæsthesia in conjunction with carcinoma or strangulated hernia.

In the ten years 1925-1934, for example, 6,741 deaths were reduced to 5,398, a reduction of 1,345, or almost exactly 20 per cent. As these deaths had actually occurred I saw no point in drawing another curve on the chart to show what it would look like if they had not happened. After all, one of the objects of this long and laborious investigation was to try and find out how many deaths had actually taken place during a century of anæsthesia.

The total deaths in England and Wales for the hundred years were 24,378, as nearly as can be ascertained. This is certainly an under-estimate. There is the fallacy mentioned above, by which all the figures before 1911 were too small, by perhaps 20 per cent.; and it is anybody's guess how many deaths took place in which anæsthesia was not mentioned on the death certificate when it should have been. This is no fault of the official statisticians. It is death certificates alone, in this instance, which are the fodder of the Registrar General. He is not responsible for what is written on them. Again, during the 1914-18 War, deaths among non-civilians were not included in the reports, whereas during the 1940-45 War they were included. This must have been due to the advances in modern civilisation which, in effect, put old men, women and children into the front line. In the next war it will be the turn of the unborn babies. The one after that is likely to be fought with bows and arrows, so there will be a return to the old method of killing off the fittest men only.

As the chart showed a welcome decline in the total deaths from the maximum of 916 in 1938 to 751 in 1946—the last year of the first century of anæsthesia—I continued it, as a matter of interest, for a few years longer in order to see whether the decline continued. The net result was that they had fallen by over 200 a year by 1949, and had reached the level of twenty years before. Considering the increasing severity and duration of operations this appears to be a notable achievement.

My opinions on this point may not be very reliable, because I have not been inside an operating theatre for fifteen years. As an anæsthetist I am obsolete, so I speak subject to correction. Three important changes have taken place since the peak year of 1938, when 916 deaths took place —the widespread and easy availability of blood transfusion, which came into being as a nation-wide service to meet the emergency of the war, the introduction of relaxants combined with light anæsthesia during the war, and, perhaps most important of all, the widespread availability of trained anæsthetists. This was greatly assisted and accelerated by the National Health Service from 1948, though it was gaining ground before this. There may be other causes, but I must leave this to be debated by more up-to-date anæsthetists.

The growth and expansion of surgery

Having at last completed my graph of anæsthetic deaths for England and Wales during the whole century (or as near as was possible to do so), I realised at once that it was very little use by itself. It merely showed a very rapidly rising curve, which could easily give a false impression. Unless it is accompanied by a similar graph showing the numerical increase in surgical operations it could be interpreted as proving that anæsthesia is becoming very much more dangerous.

The second curve on the chart is an attempt to clarify this point. I decided to go through the Annual Reports of one large, typical teaching hospital for the whole period. Naturally I chose the General Infirmary at Leeds. It was near at hand, it was old established (1767) so that its life did at least more than cover the period in question, and it has always had a high surgical reputation. I assumed that its statistics, if they were available, would be a fairly reliable index of the progress and expansion of surgery in general. By the courtesy of Mr. Fuller, Deputy House Governor, I was allowed to borrow the available reports. Unfortunately they only went back to 1873. Mr. Fuller suggested that, as a copy of the Annual Report was now always sent to the Leeds Municipal Library, it was just possible that they might also have the earlier ones. On enquiry they had some of them, so I was enabled to carry the figures back as far as 1860. Prior to that there was no information available.

The early reports are of extreme shortness and simplicity. In 1860 the total number of operations performed was 179, with 12 deaths; the average per year for the decade 1860-69 was 279 with about 24 deaths. They were mostly minor surgery by today's standards, for operations were almost entirely confined to the surface of the body. Amputations were almost the only major operations of those days, but they were relatively frequent, because amputation was the standard treatment for all compound fractures. In the first six years there were 223 amputations out of 1,533 operations, or 14 per cent. of the whole, with a mortality of 24 per cent., which was about the average. (By contrast, in the year

1925, taken at random, the amputation figures had fallen to 1·08 per cent. of the total operations.) A few lithotomies and a very occasional ovariotomy were just about the only occasions on which a body cavity was opened.

In the seven pre-Listerian years 1861-1867 there was a total of 19 ovariotomies, rather less than three a year, with not very encouraging results, for 14 of them died, or 73 per cent.

In 1925 abdominal operations, of a severity, scope and complexity undreamt of in the early days, formed 23 per cent. of all operations—1,754 out of 7,387. Their death rate was 11·6 per cent. In extracting these figures I excluded all hernias and kidney operations from the abdominals. If these, especially the hundreds of routine hernia repairs, had been included, the death rate would, of course, have been very much lower.

There are many sources of error in these operating lists. The figures given in the reports referred to the number of operations, and may not be an exact record of the number of anæsthetics; in the early days many minor operations would no doubt be done without anæsthesia at all. Again, the statistical tables were compiled by a constantly changing series of house surgeons, who were no doubt busy and harassed young men who regarded this paper work as a bore and a waste of valuable drinking time. The care and accuracy with which they were drawn up is an unknown and variable quantity, but such as they are they are the only evidence available. The detailed figures for some years were missing altogether, and the arrangement of the figures varied considerably. It was not always certain whether all operations—on out-patients, for example—were included or not. The curious dip in the curve for 1906-1909 is almost certainly accounted for in this way.

This graph is certainly not put forward as infallible or of impeccable accuracy. All that can be said is that I have tried, in the face of many difficulties, to give a true picture of the situation, as far as the figures allowed, and that the resultant curve does give some idea of the trend of surgery and its dramatic expansion. It must be remembered that I am not comparing two similar things. I am comparing deaths for a country with the expansion of surgery at one hospital only; this alone would make statisticians shudder with horror.

Thoracic and cerebral surgery was practically non-existent until comparatively late in the period. There were a few trephinings for compound fractures of the skull—57 altogether in the 18 years from 1873-1890, or 3 a year, with 20 deaths. Chest surgery was confined to the drainage of empyemata. In the same period there were 72 of these—4 per year—with 11 deaths.

Owing to a gap in the detailed reports, which extends from 1911 to 1923, it is not possible to trace the rise of these branches accurately. In 1924 and 1925 the numbers were just beginning to rise as thoracoplasty came into use. The first neurosurgeon was appointed in 1938 and the first thoracic surgeon in 1941.

In 1896 the three first anæsthetists were appointed; others were added from time to time until there were eight in 1910. Resident anæsthetists were first appointed in 1936.

If there was any peculiarity about Leeds surgery it was the fact that ether was more largely used there than in most hospitals at that time. Occasionally figures of anæsthetics given appeared in the reports. In 1892 ether was used in 66 per cent. of cases (1,566), chloroform and mixtures and sequences containing chloroform in 33 per cent. (544).

These sporadic records of the number of anæsthetics given do not tally with the numbers of operations. No doubt many anæsthetics were given in the wards and were not entered in the operating theatre books.

At this stage I passed over what I had written to Nan, with the remark that the figures were so scrappy and incomplete that I was a little disappointed. All that I had been able to do, after much hard work, was to form some sort of estimate of the total deaths in the whole century and a very rough idea—from one hospital only—of the growth of surgery.

Nan, the perfectionist, read it and said, "What you want is some more figures about the growth of surgery."

"Are you suggesting, woman," I said in strangled tones, "that I should go through a hundred years of annual reports for every hospital in the country? You know very well that I am prepared to devote unlimited time to these essays, but that would not require time—it would need eternity!"

References

[1] Census (1851). England and Wales, and Scotland.
[2] Henry M. Lyman (1882). *Artificial Anaesthesia and Anaesthetics.* London: Sampson Low.
[3] *Brit. med. J.* (1868), June 13. 591.
(1870), Mar. 12. 269.
(1872), June 15. 648.
(1880), Dec. 11. 935.
[4] *Brit. med. J.* (1891), Apr. 25. 920.
[5] John Glaister and John Glaister, Jr. (1931). *Text book of Medical Jurisprudence and Toxicology,* 5th ed. Edinburgh: Livingstone.
[6] John Glaister and John Glaister, Jr. (1931). *Text book of Medical Jurisprudence and Toxicology,* 5th ed. Edinburgh: Livingstone.
[7] *Lancet* (1908), Mar. 31. 851.
[8] *Brit med. J.* (1872), Oct. 26. 472.
[9] *Brit. med. J.* (1883), Apr. 7. 677.
[10] *Lancet* (1899), June 17. 1649.
[11] Wm. Squire (1882). *Lancet,* Oct. 14. 649.
[12] *Brit. med. J.* (1871), July 8. 33.
[13] *Lancet* (1872), Nov. 9. 690.
[14] *Lancet* (1853), Mar. 26. 307.
[15] *Brit. med. J.* (1895), Apr. 20. 891.
[16] *Lancet* (1880), Jan. 3. 2.
[17] *Brit. med. J.* (1880), Jan. 31. 178.
[18] *Brit. med. J.* (1884), May 17. 966.
[19] *Brit. med. J.* (1883), May 19. 978.
[20] *Brit. med. J.* (1870), Oct. 1. 356.
[21] *Brit. med. J.* (1871), July 29. 124.
[22] *Brit. med. J.* (1896), June 20. 1522.
[23] *Brit. med. J.* (1882), Nov. 18. 994.
[24] *Brit. med. J.* (1898), Mar. 12. 704.
[25] *Lancet* (1876), Jan. 1. 11.
(1884), Nov. 8. 848.
[26] *Lancet* (1893), Aug. 26. 482.
[27] *Lancet* (1892), July 9. 115.
[28] *Brit. med. J.* (1882), June 24. 952.
[29] *Lancet* (1891), Sept. 26. 737.
[30] *Brit. med. J.* (1894), Oct. 20. 877.
[31] *Brit. med. J.* (1894), Sept. 29. 726.
[32] *Lancet* (1854), May 20. 534.
[33] *Brit. med. J.* (1861), Nov. 16. 546.
[34] *Lancet* (1923), Feb. 10. 285.
[35] John Glaister and John Glaister, Jr. (1931). *Text book of Medical Jurisprudence and Toxicology,* 5th ed. Edinburgh: Livingstone.
[36] *Brit. med. J.* (1913), June 21. 1333.
[37] *Lancet* (1862), Dec. 20. 687.
[38] *Lancet* (1899), Sept. 23. 829.
[39] *Brit. med. J.* (1885), Jan. 31. 218.
[40] *Lancet* (1883), Jan. 6. 38.
[41] *Brit. med. J.* (1878), Oct. 19. 591.
[42] *Brit. med. J.* (1926), Oct. 9. 645.

CHAPTER 3

THE RENAISSANCE OF CHLOROFORM

Progress—Forwards or Backwards?

"The researches of antiquarians have already thrown much darkness on the subject, and it is probable, if they continue, that we shall soon know nothing at all."—Mark Twain.

When investigating the grand total of anæsthetic deaths for the whole hundred years[1] it was pointed out that chloroform appeared to have been falling out of use gradually ever since 1918, in spite of all its advantages. Before that date it was used in 75-100 per cent. of all the fatal cases; from that date there was a steady decline in the percentage, which finally reached an all time low level of 2·3 per cent. in 1949, which is as far as my chart goes. It appeared, as far as this evidence went, that chloroform was almost dead.

Its life had been prolonged for many decades by absence of reliable statistics, by dogmatic and misleading statements, by the scarcity of competitors and their shortcomings and defects, and by its own advantages. Its competitors are now, of course, much more numerous than ever before, so that it is much easier to do without it.

Its treachery, its unpredictability and its dangers—or some of them—were for a long time minimised or concealed altogether. The only one which could not in the nature of things be hidden was its liability to cause occasional sudden deaths. The cause of this was obscure and debatable; by many it was attributed to overdosage, in spite of the induction deaths which took place in a few seconds, long before any appreciable amount of the drug had been absorbed. Edward Lawrie, for example, was so concerned with the question of overdose and how to avoid it (which, according to him, was easy enough so long as his infallible method was followed), that he refused to admit that there were any other dangers at all. A further peril was that deaths were rare enough to create a false sense of security.

One of the dangers, delayed chloroform poisoning, was so rare and so slow in action that it passed practically unnoticed and unrecognised for forty-seven years. Leonard Guthrie's first article describing it was not published until 1894.[2] It took him seven years to collect his first

10 cases, in spite of being in a particularly favourable situation for their occurrence, namely in a Children's Hospital. More than nine years went by before he could report 4 more cases.[3]

A book was published in 1951, however,[4] which appears to advocate the revival of chloroform as an anæsthetic. This is strictly outside my hundred year period, but the history of the whole hundred years itself has such a direct and practical bearing on this matter that the book must be considered in some detail.

Ralph Waters conceived the novel idea that chloroform should be re-examined as though it was an entirely new anæsthetic, recently discovered. This investigation was to be carried out as a sort of centenary celebration of its first use in 1847. A vast amount of work was done at the famous Madison (Wisconsin) school of anæsthesia, so much that the book was not in fact published until four years after the centenary. It is a small volume of 124 pages, but it is full of concentrated meat. It represents a long investigation carried out over eight years by a team of about forty people, many of them anæsthetists, but with a plentiful sprinkling of other experts, including cardiologists, chemists, bio-chemists, pharmacologists and electro-cardiographers. As such it is entitled to respectful consideration.

It would be presumptuous for a long retired and obsolete anæsthetist to criticise from a technical angle the patient work of the Wisconsin school. I am no judge of the reliability of the complicated and time-consuming laboratory methods which were used so lavishly; but I have delved into the history of the subject very deeply, and there may be something to learn from this.

Generally speaking, the broad strategy of a subject does not alter throughout the course of history, whereas tactical details are constantly changing. Hannibal's campaigns well over two thousand years ago can be studied with advantage by modern generals who are wise enough to sit at the feet of the greatest master-strategist of them all. They can adjust the tactical details to modern requirements and modern weapons for themselves; but the broad principles never change. They can substitute armoured fighting vehicles driven by petrol engines for Hannibal's A.F.V.'s, which were trained elephants; they can substitute tactical air support for his diabolically clever manoeuvre at Lake Trasimeno.[5] On the 21st of June, B.C. 217, a Roman army of 40,000 men, seeking to cut off their opponents, fell into a trap themselves by marching along a lake-side road. Hannibal promptly sent detachments to seal off both ends of the road at points where a few men could hold back many times their own number. Then the rest of Hannibal's army, which was up on the heights above the lake in full, clear visibility, attacked all along the flank of the Romans, who were struggling blindly along in a dense, low-lying mist, pent up between the hills and the lake-shore. No doubt the bulk of the softening-up process was done with the natural ammunition to hand—and hundreds of tons of rocks and boulders were rolled down the steep slopes on to the unfortunates below, who were unable to see them coming through the mist until too late. There was no aiming problem. The Carthaginians could not miss such a target, even if they could not see it. It would be a target well over five miles long, if the men were marching in fours.

By ten o'clock in the morning, when the sun had cleared away the fog, the shattered remains of the disciplined Roman army were nothing but a broken and panic-stricken mob. Under any ordinary conditions they could fight, and fight well, but this was mere slaughter by unseen hands and an unseen brain. The 15,000 survivors were taken prisoner, while Hannibal's loss was negligible. Modern troops who have struggled vainly under overwhelming air attack have felt exactly the same utter impotence and helplessness. I have no doubt whatever that this was not mere luck on the part of the Carthaginian general. He was far too consistently brilliant and successful to rely on chance. I am quite sure that his intelligence officer, Carthalo, had found out that the mist was there every morning, and that his preliminary moves had forced the Romans to take that road and no other.

General George S. Patton, Jr.,[6] one of the most successful leaders of modern times, took practical lessons from history. Listen to what he says in his diary before the Normandy invasion:

> "I also read *The Norman Conquest,* by Freeman, paying particular attention to the roads William the Conqueror used in his operations in Normandy and Britanny. The roads used in those days had to be on ground which was always practicable. Therefore, using those roads, even in modern times, permits easy by-passing when the enemy resorts, as he always does, to demolition."

This, then, was one of the reasons for the lightning speed of Patton's Third Army. The fact that mechanised tanks had replaced armoured men on heavy horses made no difference whatever to general principles. Both of them needed dry ground and were useless if they were bogged down. The passage of nearly nine hundred years had left this essential unchanged. Incidentally, the Third U.S. Army liberated me from bondage, for which I am eternally grateful. I did not know at the time that their General had taken hints from William the Conqueror.

Strategically chloroform also remains unchanged. Its dangers are still there, because neither chloroform nor the human body have altered in the last hundred years. But history has at least charted the rocks and shoals for us and we know where they are. If chloroform is carelessly used, or even used carefully in the old manner unnecessary deaths will again occur. That is absolutely certain. Tactically it may be possible to overcome all dangers by modern methods, in which case the natural advantages of the drug will never allow it to die.

The Wisconsin Book

Part I is devoted to the effect of chloroform on hepatic function. It was concluded that, presuming a free airway and adequate oxygenation, its effects did not tally with statements in the literature. This was deduced from animal experiments and from function tests on patients. On page 21 it is stated that no instance of delayed chloroform poisoning occurred in 121 patients. But it had been previously said that only 65 of these actually had chloroform, the others being controls.

I have no figures for the incidence of this condition in the old days, but it was very rare, so rare that it was not even recognised in this country until chloroform had been in use for forty-seven years; and chloroform was used in almost every case at that time. To draw conclusions from its non-occurrence in 65 cases is a very vulnerable and fragile argument, especially as the cases were mostly malignant disease, which in effect means adults, the class of patient least likely to suffer from this condition. In the Essay which deals with delayed poisoning,[7] I find that I have mentioned, excluding doubtful cases, 85 patients, and 82 of them were children. If the figures had been 65,000 instead of 65 cases I would admit that a *prima facie* case had been made out for further investigation.

My doubts as to the validity of the Wisconsin conclusions about delayed chloroform poisoning, doubts which were raised by the use of a minute number of cases being alleged to prove the absence of a rare condition, were somewhat strengthened by a recent article[8] by W. M. Jones, G. Margoulis and C. R. Stephen.

> Conclusions regarding toxicity to the liver which are based on the results of liver function tests are open to question because of the lack of specificity and accuracy of function reflected by such tests. . . . All drugs demonstrated at least minimal toxicity. Chloroform was the most toxic, ethyl ether the least

toxic. Frank necrosis was observed with chloroform and vinyl ether only. Fluothane produced liver cell injury which was manifested as a fatty infiltration without necrosis.

Part II.—It was found that chloroform had no appreciable effect on renal function. So far as my historical researches go I do not think that chloroform was ever accused of this, even by its worst enemies. There was a time when ether was held to be contra-indicated in renal cases, largely because of one observation:[9]

> Many years ago, when operating upon a case of vesico-vaginal fistula, Mr. Lawson Tait observed that as the ether was pushed, the secretion of urine, by the trickling of which he was able to make out the position of the aperture, ceased, and he was obliged to change the anæsthetic to chloroform in order to complete the operation. He sent a note of the circumstances to the medical press, and pointed out that it indicated that ether suppressed the function of the kidneys, and that therefore it is a dangerous anæsthetic in cases of kidney disease.

In a recent article (1958) on bio-chemical disturbances associated with anæsthesia J. D. Robertson and S. C. Frazer of Edinburgh,[10] confirm this observation of Tait's:

> . . . with ether or cyclopropane there is a marked fall in urine flow, beginning almost immediately after the start of induction of anæsthesia and returning to nearly normal levels when consciousness returns.

They also say:

> Chloroform is a notorious hepatotoxic agent, the characteristic lesion in acute chloroform poisoning being centri-lobular necrosis.

Fluothane and Fluoromar do not appear to resemble chloroform in this way. History can tell us nothing about these newer anæsthetics, which were unknown during the first hundred years, but I am not convinced that modern work has entirely robbed chloroform of its dangerous possibilities.

Part III.—The effect of chloroform on the cardio-vascular system had been examined for ten years in the Wisconsin laboratories during a critical evaluation of other anæsthetics. Chloroform was chosen for comparison as the most toxic control agent. Two human cases were reported during the centenary investigations in which there were very narrow escapes from death. In one of them the heart actually stopped, but was re-started.

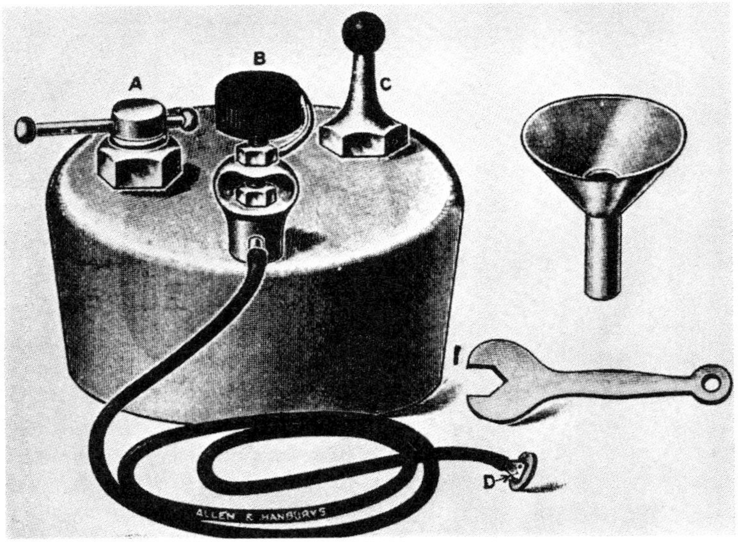

PLATE VII

Lancet, 1921, Feb. 12. 336. Warm ether bomb. S. R. Wilson and K. B. Pinson. Manchester. Advantages: 1, Self delivery, no bellows; 2, Simple and portable; 3, Unbreakable; 4, Accurate control, by needle valve; 5, Stronger vapour can be obtained; 6, Can be used with any mask or apparatus; 7, Can be used for animals. Holds ten ounces of ether. Tested to 250 lb. pressure. Screw plug for filling. Needle valve for regulating the flow of vapour. Temperature under mask 90-98 ° F. In use for 3½ years. Made by Condensed Gas Co., Manchester.

Brit. med. J., 1923, Oct. 6. 615. Improved model. Illustration taken from Allen & Hanbury's Catalogue, 1930.

This was a forerunner of machines like the Oxford Vapouriser No. 2, in that it was capable of giving off a very high percentage of ether. It was made of steel, nickel-plated, capable of withstanding a high pressure. (Ether in a closed space at a temperature of 100° C. is at a pressure of 97 lb. per square inch.) Liquid ether expands as the temperature rises, and as liquids are very incompressible, room must be left for this expansion. A special filling plug (A) is fitted which ensures that this space is left. A safety valve (C) prevents any possibility of a burst. The bomb is for use with ether only. The filler plug A must be kept screwed up tightly when in use, to prevent leakage. To fill, take out the filler plug and pour in ether until it begins to run over. If the container is hot, immerse it in cold water before unscrewing the filler plug. Turn off the valve (B) and place the whole apparatus in a large bowl of boiling water, which may cover it completely. The valve top (B) is graduated, the largest red dot marking the "off" position. The pointer is set to the zero dot when the valve is shut. This setting is adjustable, to allow for wear. If the valve gets loose tighten the gland-nut—the little nut in the centre of the valve. The small attachment (D) can be inserted through the layers covering an open mask and secured with a safety pin. To induce open the valve very slowly and gradually increase up to 40 on the dial, according to requirements. For maintenance 8-10 on the scale is sufficient. When the water cools down add fresh boiling water, shutting down the valve to some extent to compensate for the increase of pressure.

Whether it was *post hoc* or *propter hoc* the use of this bomb, mainly in Manchester at first, was followed by an epidemic of cases of ether convulsions, many of which occurred in this district about 1926. It was suggested that the hot ether vapour was a possible cause, but many cases occurred later in other places and in cases in which the bomb had not been used.

SOME EARLY PERCENTAGE CHLOROFORM INHALERS
PLATES VIII, IX, X

PLATE VIII

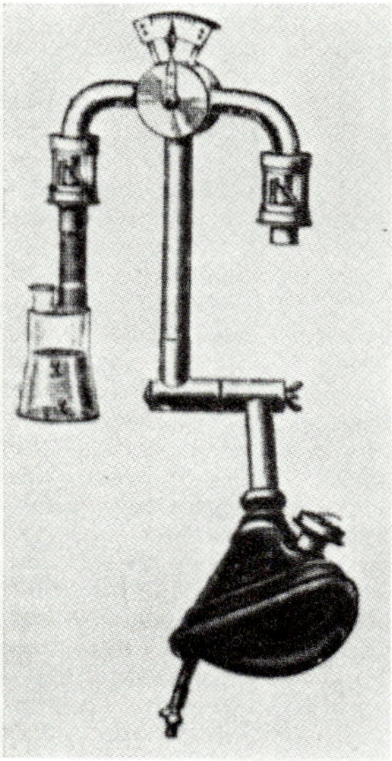

PLATE VIII

Med. Rec. N.Y., 1905, Oct. 14. Vernon Harcourt's percentage chloroform inhaler. From an article by James T. Gwathmey. The apparatus was designed by Professor A. G. Vernon Harcourt, who demonstrated it to the Society of Anæsthetists on March 6, 1903. He died August 23, 1919, in his 85th year. The inhaler was endorsed by the Chloroform Committee of the British Medical Association.

Gwathmey says that the mask was not large enough for a full inspiration, and that the valves mean increased effort, throwing a strain on the heart and lungs. Another obvious criticism is that it must have been very awkward to hold. The chloroform bottle had to be kept upright and had not to be shaken.

Brit. med. J., 1910, July 9. 47. (*Supplement*). Final Report of the Special Chloroform Committee. 52 columns. Another similar picture of the inhaler is given. The bottle is filled with chloroform to near the top of the conical part. Two coloured glass beads are dropped into it. If the temperature is below 13° C. both float; if above 15° C. both sink. In the former case less will be inhaled than the stopcock indicates, in the latter case more. The temperature should be kept between 13° and 15° by holding the bottle in the hand now and then, until the red bead floats and the blue bead begins to rise. When the pointer is at the end of the scale nearest the bottle 2% vapour is delivered. At the other end air only is given. Each small scale division equals 0·2% There is an increase tube which can be inserted into the bottle. If the larger end is put in the vapour is increased to 2·5% when the pointer is at 2; if the smaller end (marked 3%) is put in the strength is increased to 3%.

Brit. med. J., 1904, Oct. 22. 1118. Th. Hammes, Amsterdam. A modification for the Vernon Harcourt inhaler. He was satisfied with this inhaler, but found that it did not give a strong enough vapour. He used a glass tube fitted with a rubber washer. The tube was bevelled at the bottom and touched the chloroform. This gave more than 2%, but was quicker in action.

The whole point of the Vernon Harcourt inhaler was that, rightly or wrongly, 2% was thought to be safe, and the apparatus would not deliver more. If it was to be modified to give more why use the rather unwieldly thing at all?

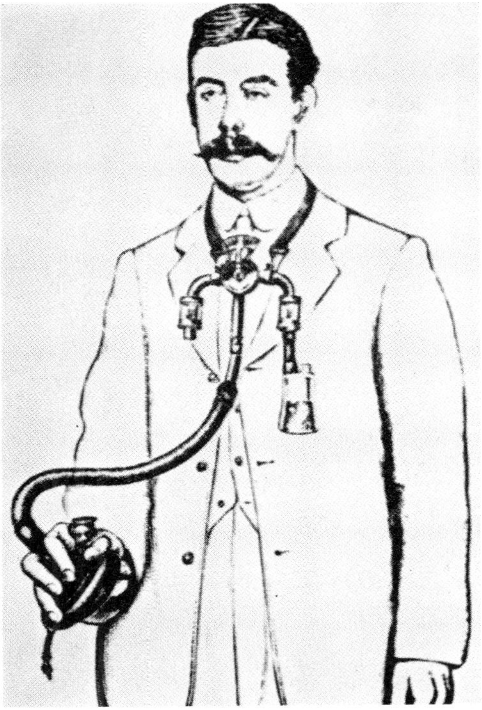

PLATE IX

Anæsthetics in Practice and Theory. J. Blomfield. 1922. London: Wm. Heinemann. A method of holding the Vernon Harcourt inhaler. It was a clumsy thing to hold. This method was not a good one, because shaking sent up the percentage.

By permission of the publishers.

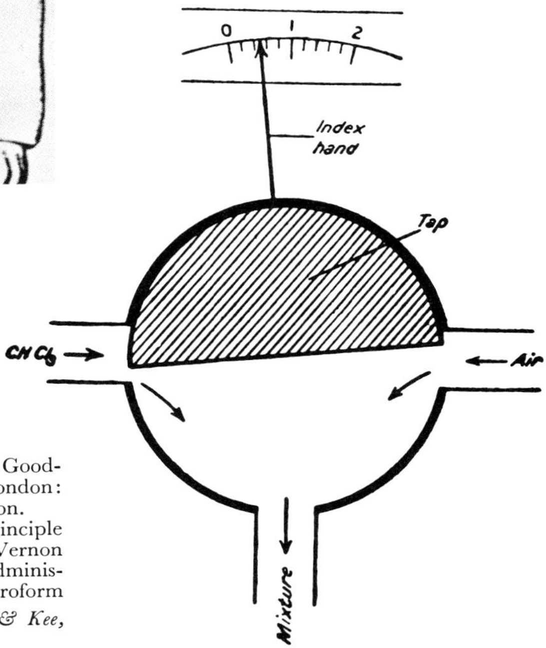

PLATE X

Chloroform Anæsthesia. A. Goodman Levy. 1922. p. 149. London: John Bale Sons & Danielsson.

Diagram showing the principle of regulating tap of the Vernon Harcourt inhaler for the administration of percentage chloroform

By permission of Macgibbon & Kee, publishers, London.

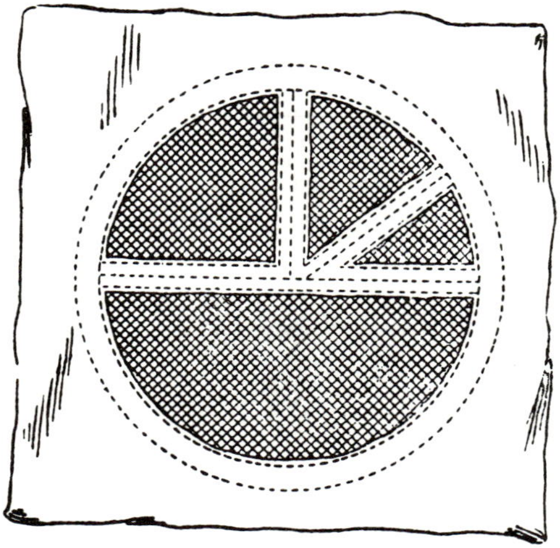

PLATE XI

Brit. med. J., 1906, Aug. 4. 247. A. G. Levy. Late Anæsthetist to Guy's Hospital. A mask cover for percentage chloroform. The shaded part represents domette sections which are sewn into a groundwork of batiste cloth. The diameter of the circle is 11 cm., and the four sections represent roughly estimated *maximum* percentage values as follows: 0·8, 1·5, 2·3, and 3·5 per cent.

A similar picture is given in Levy's book *Chloroform Anæsthesia.* 1922. London: John Bale Sons & Danielsson. It is here stated that the diamater of the circle is 4 inches and that the sections, when wetted thoroughly with chloroform and the mask fits the face closely, give 0·4, 0·8, 1·6 and 3·2 per cent. respectively.

(*This is the picture reproduced here, by permission of Macgibbon & Kee, Publishers, London.*)

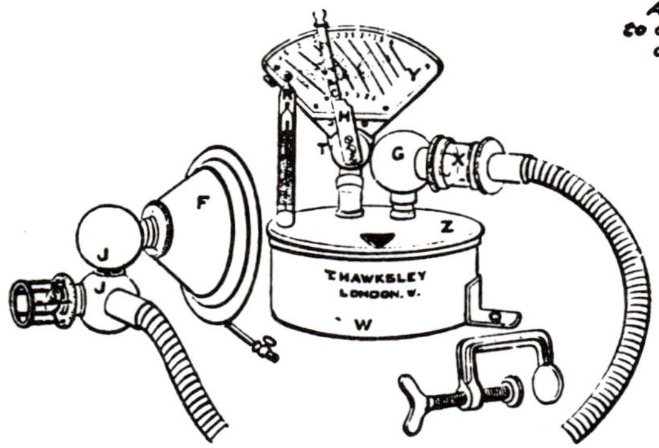

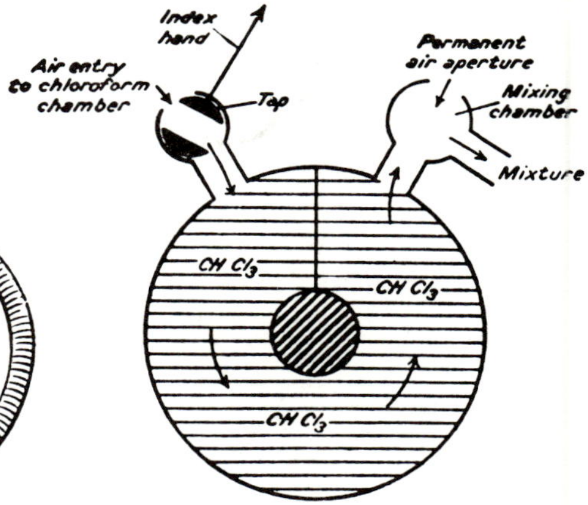

PLATES XII and XIII

Chloroform Anæsthesia. A. Goodman Levy. 1922. pp. 149. London: John Bale Sons & Danielsson.

Levy's percentage chloroform inhaler. F, Facepiece; JJ, Double junction, between facepiece and tube; S, Expiratory valve; X, Glass chamber containing inspiratory valve; G, Mixing chamber with air aperture (not shown). Z, Cover containing chloroform chamber; W, Water bath; R, Thermometer; T, Tap regulating chloroform supply (inlet not shown); H, Index hand; Y, Percentage scale.

Diagram showing the course of the air currents in Levy's inhaler. The regulating tap controls that current only which passes over the chloroform.

By permission of Macgibbon & Kee, Publishers, London.

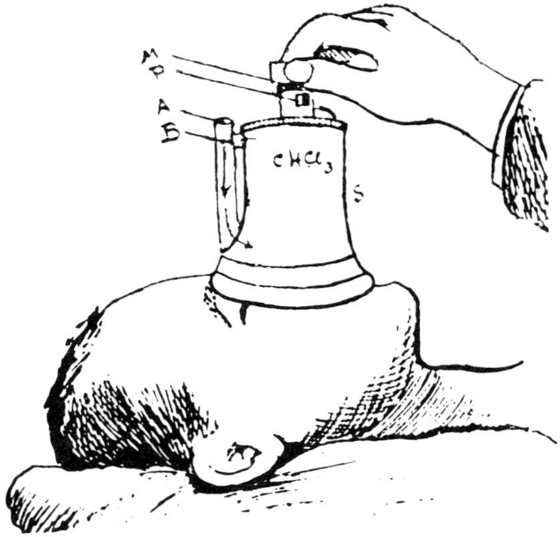

PLATE XIV

Lancet, 1916, May 13. 1003. A. D. Waller. Apparatus for chloroform anæsthesia in military practice. A modification of Prof. Reynier's. The French model delivers 0·8-2·4% chloroform vapour in air. This variation is obtained by altering the size of a small aperture through which chloroform vapour is drawn into the main air-stream. The air inlet is kept constant. It is like a carburettor. The French graduation is illusory. The dimensions have been altered. Lamp wick is used. At 2% the warming by expired air and the cooling by evaporation balance each other. The normal range is 1-2% for military use, 3% being the upper limit. Partition S separates the chloroform chamber (*above*) from the rest of the apparatus. Air is inspired through A, plus chloroform vapour through the lateral hole B. Port P is opened and closed by M and varies the dosage. 1 oz. of chloroform is poured on to the lamp-wick lining. Used at the Royal Herbert Hospital in over 2,000 cases.

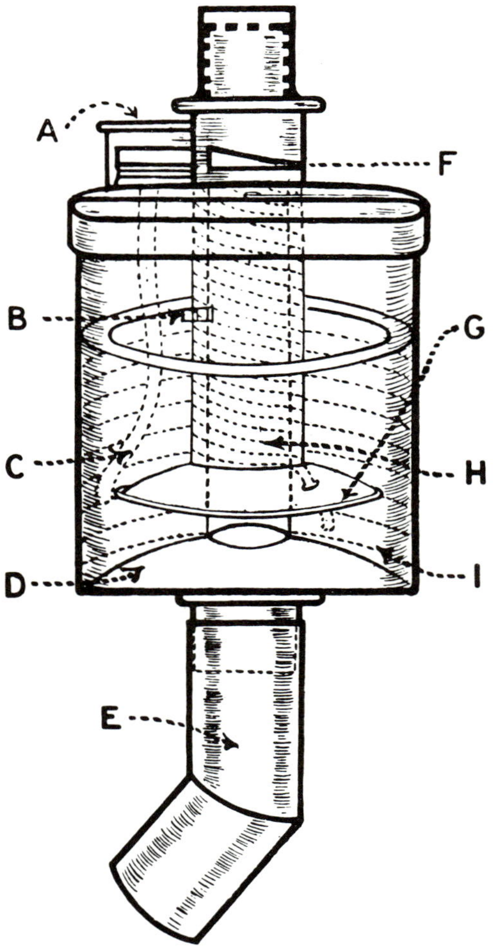

PLATE XV

Lancet, 1916, Apr. 1. 730. Charles T. W. Hirsch. Simple percentage chloroform inhaler. The principle was originally Parisian, and was introduced to this country by A. D. Waller. This obviously refers to Reynier's apparatus. There is also a picture in *A Chat on Anaesthetics*, by C. T. W. Hirsch, not dated, p. 41. London: John Bale, Sons and Danielsson. *This picture is reproduced by permission of Macgibbon & Kee, publishers, London.*

A metal cylinder is divided by a thin-domed false bottom into two chambers. The lower is coned to fit an ordinary gas facepiece, and is provided with a moveable angle piece connection for use when the patient is on his face or side. A central tube passes through the lid and upper chamber, terminating in the false bottom, and conveying air directly to the facepiece. This model is easier to fit on to the face in any position, and has a freer airway than Reynier's. Made by Cliff of Well Hall, Kent. Used in over 1,000 cases. The percentages have been verified. The facepiece is attached at E. A, filler cap, F, air inlet. Absorbent wick is fitted round the inner wall of the outer chamber and round the central tube. B, chloroform by-pass to air chamber. D, hollow dome. There are two circular baffle plates G and the one above, unlettered. The hollow dome is a false bottom. The central tube is surrounded by an air-cone which is expanded over the false bottom to form a baffle plate which distributes the air equally over the chloroform. The size of the air-port F is regulated by a moveable collar on the lid. An indicator shows the percentage of chloroform. A screw-cap allows the addition of fresh chloroform. The *Lancet* account says that 6 drachms of chloroform are put in—the booklet says 12 drachms. As the air-port is opened chloroform vapour is sucked through the by-pass B as air is sucked into a bunsen burner.

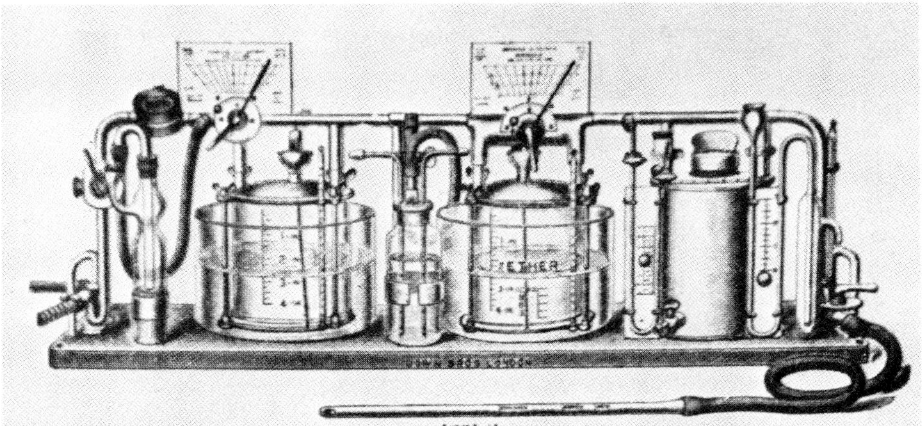

PLATE XVI

Down Bros. Catalogue. Not dated. Probably in the 1920s, when the endotracheal insufflation method was popular. Clarence Mott of Burslem. Dosimetric apparatus for chloroform, ether, gas oxygen and carbon dioxide. This is a modification of the model designed by Robert E. Kelly, of Liverpool. A flowmeter has been added to show the amount of air passing, a chloroform chamber in addition to the ether chamber, a sight feed gas and oxygen bottle similar to Boyle's and a water manometer. This gives the respiratory index in addition to the usual mercury manometer for showing the pressure of the delivered gases. There is an extra deep heating chamber. The flowmeter enables the scale of percentages to be added. Thermometers are fitted to each of the water jackets.

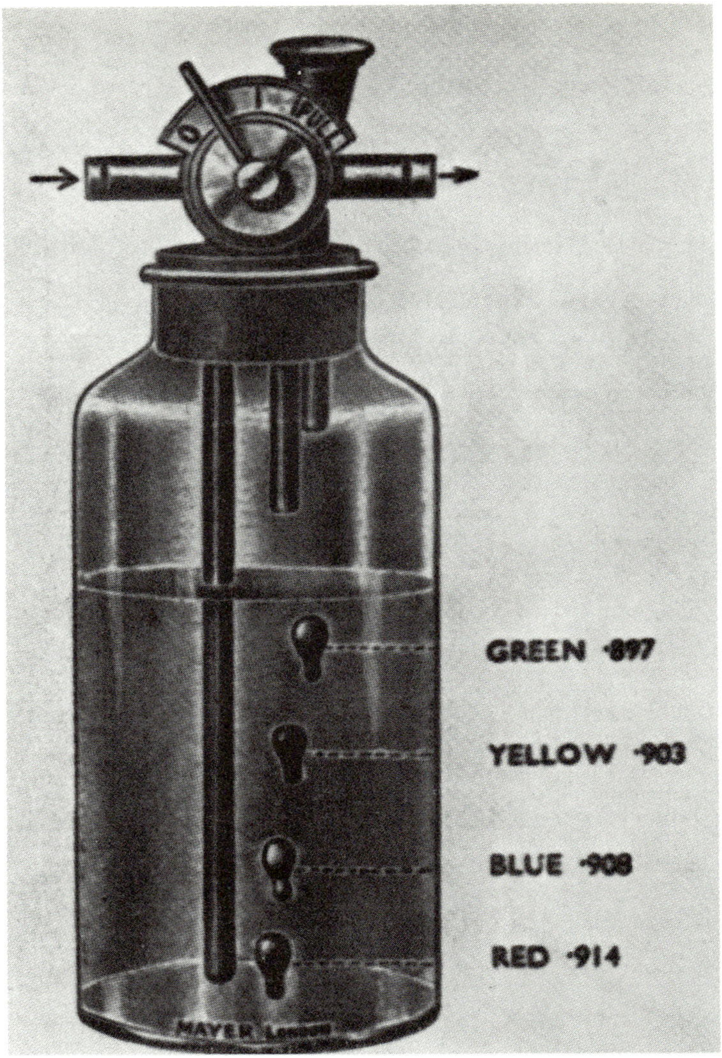

PLATE XVII

Legend—see page 49

"The occurrence of ventricular tachycardia in twenty of the fifty-two (examined for cardiac irregularities) . . . is important since cardiologists consider it to be extremely serious and frequently a precursor of ventricular fibrillation."

And yet they say that the effects of chloroform were not so bad as expected. What did they expect? Death in all cases? May I remind you of some large series of chloroform cases, some of them good, some of them bad, in order to restore a sense of proportion to the problem.

Andrews	117,078 with 43 deaths or 1 in 2,723.
Coles	152,620 with 53 deaths or 1 in 2,873.
B. W. Richardson	35,165 with 11 deaths or 1 in 3,196.
Julliard	524,507 with 161 deaths or 1 in 3,258.
Dr. Gurlt[11]	27,029 with 29 deaths or 1 in 932.
St. Bartholomew's, for the 12 years 1884-1895 inclusive[12]	22,219 with 14 deaths or 1 in 1,587.
R. Beatson Hird. General Hospital, Birmingham, 1915[13]	5,158 with 14 deaths or 1 in 368.

PLATE XVII

Theory and Practice of Anæsthesia. M. D. Nosworthy. 1937. London: Hutchinson. Rowling's percentage chloroform bottle.

S. Thompson Rowling was born in 1874. He was anæsthetist to the General Infirmary at Leeds for many years. He died October 12, 1950 in his 76th year. He designed a closed ether inhaler, a two piece airway, an automatic drop bottle and anæsthetic screen and an anæsthetic table as well as this bottle, which was the most original of his inventions. He was an enthusiastic user of chloroform, given from this device.

If the bottle contains a mixture of 6 dr. of chloroform and 12 oz. of liquid paraffin, its specific gravity is 0·914 at 70° F., and it will vapourise 3·5%. The red specific gravity bead of 0·914 will fall when the proportion of chloroform is less than this. When the bottle contains 5 dr. the mixture has a sp. gr. of 0·908 and vapourises 3%. The blue bead of sp. gr. 0·908, which has been floating, sinks when the concentration falls below this point. When 2 dr. of chloroform has been evaporated the 4 dr. in the mixture has a sp. gr. of 0·903 and will give off 2·5%. The yellow (0·903) bead will begin to sink at less than this. The green bead (0·897) will begin to sink at less than 2%.

All floating—% exceeds 3·5		3 sink —% exceeds 2·0%
1 sinks — exceeds 3·0		all sink—% less than 2·0%
2 sink —% exceeds 2·5		

The authors of this section remark, very wisely, that the final value of any laboratory research depends upon clinical proof that the results may be transferred to man. This is absolutely true, but what made them think that it was possible to obtain proof of any kind from a tiny group of cases?

Part IV.—This is a clinical evaluation of chloroform in 1,111 administrations—again a very small number when compared with the general death rate from chloroform as shown in the large lists shown above. There were no deaths in these 1,111 cases, though dangerous signs were observed in 12, or about 1 per cent. It will be noticed that several of the large clinical series did not have a death, on the average, until two or three times the Madison total had been reached.

Part V.—This section discusses the concentration of chloroform in blood and the respired air. The finding corroborates Clover's estimate of a little less than 1·5 per cent. in air very closely.

Part VI.—This is a summing up by the originator of the idea, Ralph M. Waters. Very wisely he says that the statements about absence of delayed chloroform poisoning were correct enough in the context in which they were used. I take this to mean that he realises the absurdity of drawing any conclusions at all from such a small number. "It is well known, however, that severe damage to the liver, and possibly to the kidneys also, has been known to follow the administration of chloroform. It can occur again."

He finally concludes that chloroform is the most powerful of all anæsthetics, that its speed of action lies between that of ether and cyclopropane, and that there is no reliable method of sufficiently delicate control. A lack of fine control is a temptation to overdosage; this temptation *must* be resisted. Control in steps of 0·1 per cent. is needed, which is beyond the capacity of any existing apparatus. The signs of anæsthesia are often unreliable, and light anæsthesia may be satisfactory. Chloroform does not stimulate respiration but depresses it. Changes in saturation are slow in deep anæsthesia, and any haste or impatience may easily lead to overdose. Reduction of blood pressure may be central in high concentrations, even to cardiac arrest. Given good control the blood pressure can be maintained or reduced at will. In spite of these criticisms Waters says that chloroform does not deserve to be abandoned altogether as an anæsthetic. As it is non-irritant the patient cannot protect himself against it, therefore the responsibility for overdose lies on the anæsthetist. Surely this applies to all anæsthetics, perhaps to a rather less degree?

Waters speaks with authority on a subject of this kind. It was he and his department who did the experimental and clinical work on the introduction of cyclopropane into medical practice in 1933. I was fortunate enough to see some of their impressively careful and painstaking procedure on a visit to Madison in that year. So the introduction of a new anæsthetic was no new thing to him.

But as a historian I wonder whether the history of the subject has been sufficiently considered? I would like to put forward a series of questions to be answered by anybody who proposes to use or advocate the use of chloroform. If they can answer all the questions with a 'Yes', without reserve or qualification, then it may be justifiable.

1. Will you promise not to back your arguments about the safety of chloroform (with its overall mortality of perhaps 1 in 2,000 under the old conditions) with statistics of a few hundred cases?

2. Can you guarantee, always and in all cases, to avoid overdosage, when dealing with the most powerful of all anæsthetics? You must be able to do this even at the end of a long day when you are tired, even in an emergency in the middle of the night, when you are more than tired. Can you guarantee that all who use it will remember all the time that it is eight times as strong as ether, and that it can kill anybody quickly, however strong or resistant they may be? If you rely on automatic or mechanical control, can you remember that Waters admitted that no satisfactory means of accurate control existed as late as 1951?

3. Can you guarantee that chloroform will *never*, under any circumstances (except possibly in labour cases) be used for induction? For, according to history, no amount of skill, of knowledge, of experience or even of accurate dose regulation can avoid primary cardiac failure in Occidental peoples. There is some evidence that in Orientals and in tropical conditions this danger may not exist. But it exists everywhere else and all the time—only occasionally, mind you. It is possible to induce with it many hundreds of times without danger, but sooner or later, with paralysing suddenness it will happen. The pathologist cannot find fright at the post-mortem, but fright is the determining factor in these deaths, which are particularly liable to occur in young and healthy adults, when tragedy is least expected. The only way to be certain of avoiding them is to avoid chloroform for induction, even if you are going to use it later. Don't think "it can't happen to me." It may not, for a while, but it assuredly will if you induce with chloroform long enough.

4. Can you guarantee, always and in every case, if a sudden heart failure should occur, either primary or secondary, that you can instantly restart the heart? And are you sure that it will work every time? The

old methods of artificial respiration combined with galvanic batteries hardly ever succeeded. Can you succeed where they failed? And have you thought up a good story to tell the patient who wakes up after a tonsillectomy and finds that he has also the six inch wound of a cardiac massage?

5. Can you guarantee that you have definitely guarded against the risk of delayed chloroform poisoning? The Madison workers appear to think that a free airway and adequate oxygenation may protect against this—on the evidence of 65 cases. But the condition was always a rare one. It is by no means enough to give a tentative opinion on very scanty evidence when the penalty for a wrong answer is death. Do you *know* that you can prevent it? It is no use saying that you will use small amounts only. Four drachms[14] have caused death in an adult.

Lewis Beesly's terrible statistics of 1906 should be engraved in letters of fire on every chloroform inhaler or vapouriser that is hereinafter designed.[15] They are worth repeating:

They referred to perforated appendix cases operated upon at the Royal Hospital for Sick Children, Edinburgh.

Chloroform, 19 cases, 14 deaths, with symptoms of delayed chloroform poisoning in all of them.

Chloroform ether mixtures, 3 cases, 1 death, from chloroform poisoning.

That gives a death rate of 68 per cent. for chloroform. Then a change was made to ether, and 24 cases were dealt with, with 2 deaths, not from poisoning. This was a death rate of 8·3 per cent., which was reasonable enough, considering the severity of the condition and the dangers of peritonitis in the pre-antibiotic era.

It is a rare condition, except in toxic children. No figures exist as to its frequency. Taken over all it may be even rarer than primary cardiac failure, which it resembles in another way—in that it was unpredictable, untreatable and almost inevitably fatal. Are you sure you can treat it effectively if you meet it?

When I had written this Essay thus far I thought that I had finished it: so I carried out my usual routine and handed it to Nan, my wife and helper, my valued and constructive critic. She read it and remarked, in effect, that I was sticking my neck out in writing about modern times after having been retired for fifteen years—and moreover during a period of constant change and the most rapid alterations on record. She also said that I was straying outside my one hundred year period, which was quite true but intentional; and that I knew nothing about modern anæsthesia, which was also true. As usual she had put her finger straight on to the weak spot.

The first person I wrote to in my quest for up to date information was Dr. H. G. Epstein of Oxford.[16] He thought that Waters's book on chloroform was rather unsatisfactory for various reasons, the main defect being the uncontrolled administration of chloroform in gas mixtures as described in the book. "As will be apparent from the following there would have been little difficulty for the collaborators of that book to make use of reasonably quantitative procedures." He then gave me a list of references to various percentage inhalers, most of which, however, were later in date than the book and so not available to the authors at the time the work was done.

The only one mentioned by Epstein which was available in 1951 was the E.S.O. (Epstein, Suffolk, Oxford) chloroform inhaler, designed for use by airborne troops in 1943. It was fitted with a manual thermo-compensator.

Waters had said that no vapouriser existed in 1951 which would deliver percentages accurate to 0·1. Whether or not that was the case Epstein did not think that such a degree of accuracy was necessary.

"In the first instance there is, I think, no evidence that the accuracy of an inhaler would have to be as close as 0·1% in order to get repeatable anæsthetic conditions with chloroform/air mixtures. The trouble with the work described in the book by Waters is that in most cases they had no idea at all about the inspired chloroform concentration. . . .

"Little attention is paid in the book by Waters to A. G. Levy's book on Chloroform; although various pharmacological and physiological aspects of that book are long outdated, there are a number of shrewd comments and findings on the significance of the inspired chloroform levels. The two inhalers designed and described by Levy (1904) were perhaps a little inconvenient in use, but when we calibrated the output some fourteen years ago under varying respiratory conditions, the values were reasonable accurate—I seem to remember deviations of less than 0·3 vol. per cent.

"By about 1943 the so-called E.S.O. chloroform inhaler (Epstein, Suffolk, Oxford), intended for airborne troops, had been designed and tested. Later on quite a few other people used them for quantitative work. . . .

"We never found any evidence that changes in concentration of say 0·2 vol. per cent. had any visible clinical or physiological effect. I therefore think there is little need of requiring an accuracy of 0·1 vol. per cent. from any anæsthetic inhaler . . . the famous Copper Kettle has also been used for chloroform in recent years. . . ."

This last sentence is not a valid criticism of Waters's work, for the Copper Kettle was not, I think, introduced until the year after the Wisconsin book was published.[17] The originator himself says of it:

"Potentially, a lethal concentration of ether can be introduced into the bag of a closed system, since concentration more than ten times the amount required for maintenance of anæsthesia are provided by the vaporizer. *Caution equal to that when adding cyclopropane to a closed system is indicated.*"

If this is the case with a comparatively weak anæsthetic like ether, how much more does it apply to chloroform, which is at least eight times stronger? Lucien Morris and Stanley A. Feldman in a paper on the general principles of design and function of anæsthetic vapourisers[18] refer to the present tendency towards designing machines which keep the anæsthetic liquid at a high, sometimes even a boiling point temperature. This can give a flow of theoretically 100 per cent. vapour, which is then metered and diluted before it is delivered to the patient. This may make for accuracy of control, but it leaves a loophole for easy and fatal mistakes. The authors refer to the Pinson bomb and the Oxford Vapouriser No. 2, which both used this principle . . . "with lethal consequences if there is failure of the gas flow."

The Copper Kettle was actually designed for chloroform, to obtain vernier control of vapour strength, efficiency of vaporization and moderate thermo-stability, but was largely used for ether.[19]

Deaths have occurred during the use of the Copper Kettle usually because of failure to appreciate the fundamental principles of its design. It must be realised that the outflow of vapor concentration from the vaporizer itself is lethal unless diluted, and may represent in the case of ether from 50 to 60 per cent., or even 70 per cent. concentration, depending on the temperature within the vaporizer.

. . . users of efficient vaporizers, such as the Copper Kettle, must abandon this fallacious reasoning (that ether is a safe agent in the hands of even the inexperienced) and carefully avoid misuse of this effective device.

Personally I have never even seen any of these new vaporisers, nor did I know how they worked until I looked up the references kindly given to me by Dr. Epstein. Accurate they may be—so is a loaded rifle—and both these things seem to have extremely dangerous potentialities, however safe they may be in the hands of the expert. The designers of the Copper Kettle admit that deaths have occurred—even with ether—owing to ignorance of their power.

The next person from whom I sought advice was Dr. M. H. Armstrong Davison, of Newcastle, who uses chloroform quite a lot. As he says:[20]

"Once upon a time, anæsthesia was dominated by the volatile liquid agents. With the advent of the relaxants, the former lords of narcosis fell into a position of less importance. They have managed to survive until our own day, but the future does not lie with them."

Dr. Armstrong Davison was more or less pushed into the use of chloroform, in the first instance by insistent surgeons when he was a student, and later by war-time shortages. He points out its overwhelming convenience and advantages as an inhalation anæsthetic under war conditions, which are of course undoubted.

"I almost *never* give an anæsthetic without giving 8 breaths of chloroform, rising in strength each two breaths from 0·5% to about 6%, and I have used this technique for 24 years. (It is an admirable preliminary to turning on the ether.) Yet, I do believe that my success with chloroform has been largely because I am frightened of it, or, at least, have a very healthy respect for its potency. However, these cases amount to some 30,000 at the very least, and although but little is used, it *is* used in induction, and the concentration rises to far above that which the pundits permit . . . my opinion differs from yours —but I guess I'm in a minority. . . . Yes, chloroform is dangerous and potent, but so is a motor car, and the anæsthetist who uses it, like the driver of a car, should be sufficiently skilled to neutralise the dangers."[21]

Here, then, is Counsel for the Defence, and a skilful and experienced counsel, too. As I pointed out in my reply, thanking him for his assistance, I am not opposing progress. I only want to be sure that the progress is forwards and not backwards. I still think that the historical objections to chloroform are very strong indeed. It may be that, in the hands of the expert, it will be found to be safe, as it appears to be in the hands of Dr. Davison, but will it remain in the hands of the expert?

H. W. Loftus Dale[22] commented very aptly that one of the most famous last words (for the patient) is, "Just give her a whiff, old man." And with that, some ignoramus like me, who has never seen a Copper Kettle or an Oxford Vapouriser No. 2, is told off to give a short anæsthetic for some minor operation. Knowing nothing and fearing nothing he twiddles a knob, as he might twiddle the lever of the old bubble bottle, and sends a blast of undiluted vapour into the unfortunate patient, with the inevitable result.

Another witness, D. S. Middleton[23] was compelled to use chloroform by war conditions while a Japanese prisoner of war. In two years he had 2,978 cases, 811 of them with chloroform. There was 1 death due to it. He knew of 2 other deaths from chloroform in other camps—one from syncope during induction, the other from delayed poisoning. So it appears that chloroform has not lost its potency. This reporter was not without previous experience of chloroform. He had previously given it more than 500 times with no fatalities.

John Gillies[24] found by means of a questionnaire that, out of 865 general practitioners in Scotland 94 per cent. used chloroform for obstetrics. For minor surgery 26 per cent. used chloroform or mixtures. For major surgery 53 per cent. used chloroform or mixtures. Gillies estimated that out of 1,084,870 chloroform cases the death rate in the general practitioners' cases was 1 in 7,000, in specialists' practice, who naturally got the bad risks and the severe cases, 1 in 2,760. "Occasionally one met with an engaging frankness, as in the case of the doctor who said he had given chloroform six times and three of the patients had died, since when he had given it up."

It appears, therefore, that chloroform is perhaps more used than I thought it was. The weak point of Gillies' statistics is that there was a good deal of estimation in them—words such as 'often' and 'seldom' were translated into figures, which leaves room for a very big margin of error either way.

Postscript.—At this point I really had finished the Essay, having dipped into modern literature for a change. But one thing led to another and in one of the modern articles I came across another reference which interested me enough to look it up. Karl L. Siebecker and O. Sidney Orth reported from Madison in 1956, five years after the publication of the Wisconsin book,[25] 7 chloroform cases for thoracic operations.

Of these 7 cases 4 had severe hepatic damage, 2 of them severe enough to be fatal. One was a man of fifty-seven for a lobectomy. The anæsthesia lasted 4 hours 50 minutes, chloroform being used for $2\frac{3}{4}$ hours of this time. It is not stated how much was used, unfortunately. The patient died on the third day with acute central necrosis of the liver. The other was a man of forty-eight for a segmental resection. The anæsthesia lasted 2 hours 25 minutes, during which chloroform was given for 1 hour 55 minutes. The patient died on the fourth day, with severe centrilobular necrosis of the liver and renal tubular degeneration. (He had chronic alcoholism and cirrhosis before operation.) Two other cases developed non-fatal jaundice after $1\frac{1}{2}$ hours and $\frac{1}{2}$ hour of chloroform respectively.

Examination of the anæsthesia records of both patients who received severe enough damage to cause death reveals that there were periods of hypotension and bradycardia during the administration of chloroform. These are danger signals during the administration and should be considered evidence of overdosage.

There is perhaps no one who is so universally disliked as the person who says, "I told you so." But I don't give a damn whether I am disliked or not, and I have no axe to grind. That is one of the joys of being retired. Just read the Essay again and see whether my doubts were justified or not. You will have to take my word for it that I knew nothing of these 7 cases until after the Essay was complete except for this postscript.

I leave it to others to decide the question of suboxygenation and its bearing on chloroform poisoning. The fact remains that these patients had chloroform and died of the old-fashioned chloroform poisoning just as Guthrie's children died in the 1880s. I still wonder whether we are progressing forwards or backwards.

References

[1] Sykes, W. S. (1960). *The First Hundred Years of Anæsthesia.* Vol. II, chap. 2. Edinburgh: Livingstone.

[2] *Lancet* (1894), Jan. 27. 193.
(1894), Feb. 3. 257.

[3] *Lancet* (1903), July 4. 10.
Sykes, W. S. (1960). *The First Hundred Years of Anæsthesia.* Vol. III, chap. 4. Edinburgh: Livingstone.

[4] Ralph M. Waters (1951). *Chloroform: A study after* 100 *years.* University of Wisconsin Press.

[5] Harold Lamb (1959). *Hannibal. One man against Rome,* p. 82. London: Hale.

[6] George S. Patton, Jr. (undated, probably 1946 or 1947). *War as I knew it.* London: Allen.

[7] Sykes, W. S. (1960). *The First Hundred Years of Anæsthesia.* Vol. III, chap. 4. Edinburgh: Livingstone.

[8] W. M. Jones, G. Margoulis and C. R. Stephen (1958). *Anesthesiology.* 19. 715.

[9] *Med. Ann.* (1899), 160.

[10] *Brit. med. Bull.* (1958). Vol. 14. 8.

[11] *Lancet* (1897), Dec. 25. 1671.

[12] *Brit. med. J.* (1897), Aug. 21. 500.

[13] *Brit. med. J.* (1915), Apr. 17. 698.

[14] *Lancet* (1934), Sept. 15. 597.

[15] *Brit. med. J.* (1906), May 19. 1142.

[16] Personal communication from Dr. Epstein, dated 15th July, 1960.

[17] Lucien E. Morris (1952). *Anesthesiology.* Vol. 13. 587.

[18] *Anesthesiology* (1958). Vol. 19. 642.

[19] *Anesthesiology* (1958). Vol. 19. 650.

[20] *Anæsthesia* (1959). Vol. 14. 127.

[21] Personal communication from Dr. M. H. Armstrong Davison, dated 30/7/60.

[22] *Brit. med. J.* (1946), Mar. 16. 408.

[23] *Anæsthesia* (1948). Vol. 3. 53.

[24] *Anæsthesia* (1948). Vol. 3. 45.

[25] *Anesthesiology* (1956). Vol. 17. 792.

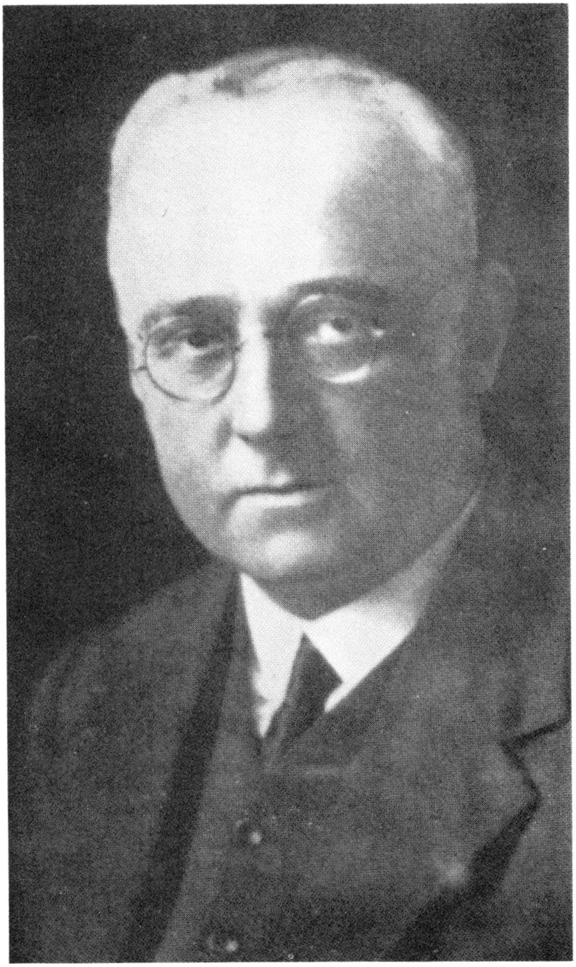

PLATE XVIII

S. THOMPSON ROWLING, M.D., F.F.A.R.C.S.
Photo by courtesy of Mrs. Rowling.

Anæsthetist to the General Infirmary at Leeds, 1906-1945.
Honorary Anæsthetist, 1946.

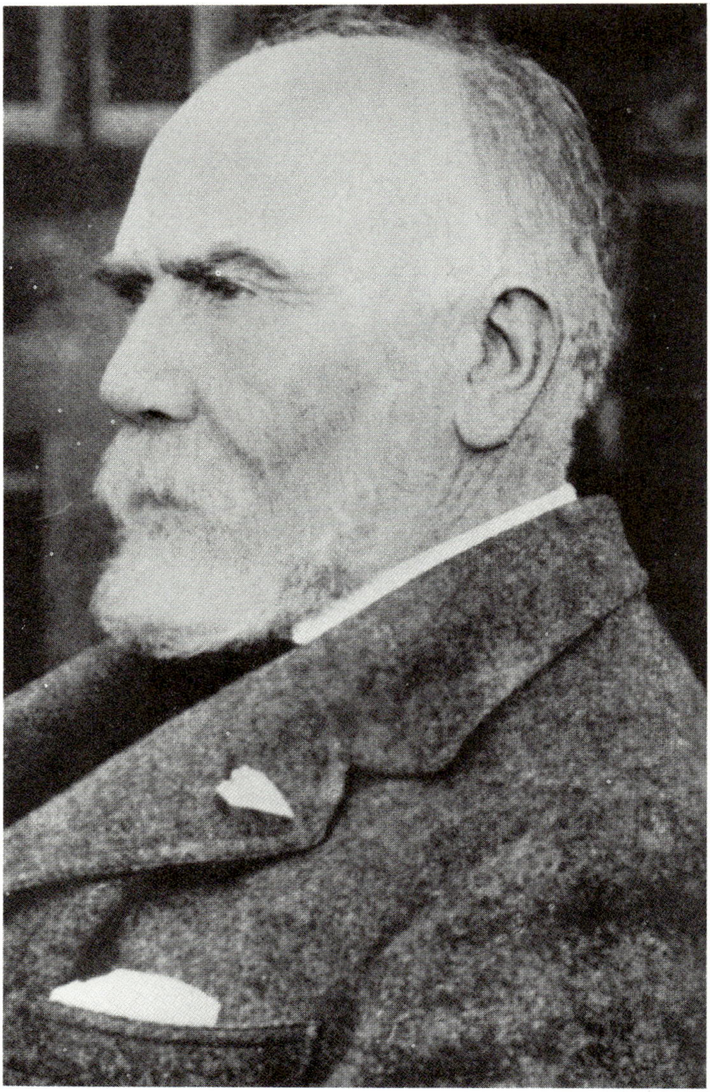

PLATE XIX

Brit. med. J., 1925, Jan. 31. 242. Sir James Mackenzie. Born 1853. Qualified at Edinburgh in 1878. In general practice in Burnley, Lancashire, for 28 years. 1907, Physician to the London Hospital. F.R.C.P. 1913. At the end of the 1918 War retired to St. Andrews to devote himself to clinical research. Died January 26, 1925. The founder of modern cardiology.

(*By permission of the Brit. med. J.*).

CHAPTER 4

ANÆSTHESIA AND THE CARDIOLOGISTS

"I found the task so truly arduous, so full of difficulties, that I was almost tempted to think . . . that the motion of the heart was only to be comprehended by God."—WILLIAM HARVEY (April 1, 1578-June 3, 1657), *De Motu Cordis et Sanguinis in Animalibus, 1628.*

As a result of a search through twelve British and American text-books on heart disease, which totalled 6,434 pages between them, I came to the surface with a feeling of deep disappointment. I was, of course, looking for information about anæsthesia in heart cases. What I found was, for the most part, vague, sketchy and of little practical use. Moreover, much of it was obsolete. In only one book out of the twelve was any serious attempt made to give an up to date survey of the subject, to the extent of fifteen pages. The other eleven, with 5,312 pages between them, devoted a total space of sixteen pages to the risks and the management of anæsthesia in cardiac cases, about 0·3 per cent. of their available space.

This scrutiny also produced an idea for a possible line of research. It is quite possible that this has been anticipated, of course, for I have been retired from anæsthesia for fifteen of its most productive and progressive years and am quite out of touch with modern developments. However, here it is, for what it is worth.

Take a young and enthusiastic anæsthetist, preferably one who has some interest in general medicine and one who can write. Let him have a few years' practical experience in the operating theatre, in order to realise to the full the extent of the problems and the vastness of the unexplored territory in front of him. Then transfer him to a cardiological department for a long enough time to learn the basic principles and methods of modern cardiology, with a guarantee against loss of seniority on his return to his own work. Then bring him back to his proper sphere, in due course, when he has accumulated more experience, to write a helpful and authoritative book on cardiology as applied to anæsthesia. The figures given above prove that there is ample room for a book of this kind; the cardiologists can't do it, because of their total ignorance of anæsthesia.

This specially trained cardiologist-anæsthetist, in addition to writing from his own experience and knowledge, might also collect the opinions and practice of other anæsthetists. He might arrange them, classify them—and, if need be, criticise them. He could investigate all the existing methods of estimating operative risk, and try out new ones of his own, for there is a lot of work to be done on this subject—important work. The whole project would be long, slow and expensive, covering at least fifteen years, but given the right man it might prove to be a valuable economy—in lives—in the long run.

There is good historical precedent for this idea. Leonard Guthrie was a chloroformist before he took up the dual appointment of physician and pathologist to a children's hospital. This varied and combined training produced spectacular results, for he was the man, above all others, who identified and described the insidious and easily missed effects of delayed chloroform poisoning in a series of patients large enough to form *prima facie* evidence of its existence. And every scrap of evidence he could produce was needed, for his theory was hotly denied by Watson Cheyne (later Sir Watson Cheyne) who could not be brought to believe that chloroform was the culprit. Cheyne was one of Lister's disciples, educated in Edinburgh and brought up to believe, as an article of faith, that chloroform was perfect in every way. The fact that he had had a death from chloroform (on the table) under his own hands had by no means shaken his belief in its harmlessness.[1] Even with all Guthrie's advantages it took him six years to collect his first 10 cases, and another nine years to add 4 more.

Now it is up to me to produce some evidence for my dissatisfaction with the cardiologists' treatment of the subject of anæsthesia. It will be convenient to take the books in chronological order. The first is that of Sir James Mackenzie, that great general practitioner who revolutionised the study of heart disease by the simple device of following up his patients for many years—which he could do in general practice, provided he was willing to work about seventeen hours a day—and which the hospital physicians could not do.

Mackenzie was born in 1853, qualified at Edinburgh in 1878 and was a family doctor in Burnley, an industrial town in the north of England, for twenty-eight years. His publications were so revolutionary, and yet so sound and unassailable, that he had a Continental reputation while he was still in general practice and before anybody in England had ever officially heard of him. But then something unique happened. His reputation grew so great that he was invited to London and appointed Physician to the London Hospital. This was in 1907. He was elected to the Fellowship of the Royal College of Physicians in 1913, and at the end of the 1914-1918 War, original to the last, he gave up his consulting practice and retired to the small Scottish university (and golf) town of St. Andrews. Here he founded an Institute for Clinical Research, for he believed, from his own experience, that general practice in a more or less static community was a most fertile field for research. He died on January 26th, 1925.

His book on the diagnosis and treatment of heart disease[2] was published in 1916. It devotes one and a half pages out of 248 to anæsthesia. He admits that his experience has been entirely confined to chloroform.

> "In some hospitals there are no deaths in 20,000 cases of chloroform anæsthesia, in others there is a death in every two or three thousand. This would seem to suggest some fault in administration rather than in the drug. . . ."

Most of Mackenzie's work was original, but here he was on ground which was strange, and to him quite uninteresting. He was, of course, merely paraphrasing Syme's famous lecture of 1855. He was only two years old when this lecture was delivered, but it had passed into history as an almost indestructible legend.

Syme's simple assumption, which was the foundation of the whole myth, was that as there had been up to that time 13 deaths in London and only 1 in Edinburgh, the London death rate was thirteen times higher, therefore the London men knew thirteen times less about chloroform than Syme did. He had the infallible method, founded on a far too small series of cases, and kindly offered to teach them. What he completely and conveniently forgot, or ignored, was the fact that the death rates were exactly equal, if one considered the relative population of the two towns.

The persistence of Syme's faulty assumptions is well illustrated here. They still conditioned and contaminated Mackenzie's first class brain no less than sixty-one years later. Of course, his interest was primarily in heart disease, not in anæsthesia. If it had chanced to be the other way round his original and iconoclastic intellect would soon have detected the fallacy.

Mackenzie was on firmer ground—ground which he had made for himself on solid foundations—when he gives his own opinions, although they are somewhat vague.

> "If there is a good or fair response to effort I unhesitatingly give consent to the use of the anæsthetic, no matter what the organic lesion may be . . ." and "the guide should always be the state of the heart muscle and its efficiency (in) response to effort."

Herein lay the secret of the advances he had made in cardiology. Every since Laennec first introduced the stethoscope physicians had been fascinated by it and had devoted themselves to identifying, distinguishing and classifying the various forms of heart murmurs. This became a very learned, but rather arid, subject, for hospital physicians got few opportunities of following up their cases, with the result that little was known about the real importance or prognostic significance of the murmurs. The only cases which were effectively followed up were those which died in hospital. (The post-mortem reports, in bound volumes, at St. Bartholomew's Hospital used to be euphemistically and significantly labelled "Register of Complete Cases.")

The natural result was that heart murmurs assumed a tremendous and altogether too gloomy importance. The patients who lived and went back to work again dropped out of sight altogether, except to the seeing eyes of a general practitioner of genius, like Mackenzie. As far as the hospital was concerned they were merely Incomplete Cases, who had most unfairly cheated the knife of the pathologist.

Mackenzie, therefore, came to lay stress on the presence or absence of heart failure, and on the cardiac response to effort, as being more important than valvular murmurs as such. He also distinguished between the unimportant and the dangerous changes of rhythm by recording them both and waiting—for years if necessary—to see which arrhythmias killed the patient and which did not. He used a polygraph ink recorder, the precursor of the electrocardiograph, but always stressed the fact that instruments were not the only, not even the most important part of his method.

He does not mention status lymphaticus at all in his book, although at the time he wrote it was the reputed cause of many deaths under anæsthesia—and nobody doubted its existence at that time, as they did in later years.

The next book on my list is a combined British and American production.[3] It contains 491 pages, long enough, one would think, to be comprehensive, and yet at this time, in 1942, anæsthesia and its ominous enemy status lymphaticus are not mentioned at all.

The third book (1948) was American.[4] It had 598 pages, two of which were devoted to surgery and anæsthesia. They are vague and sketchy, and of little use to an anæsthetist faced with a difficult heart problem. "The use of curare will be considered," says the author, but does not say how it should be considered, whether as a milestone of progress or a tombstone. Cyclopropane is ignored, with all its special

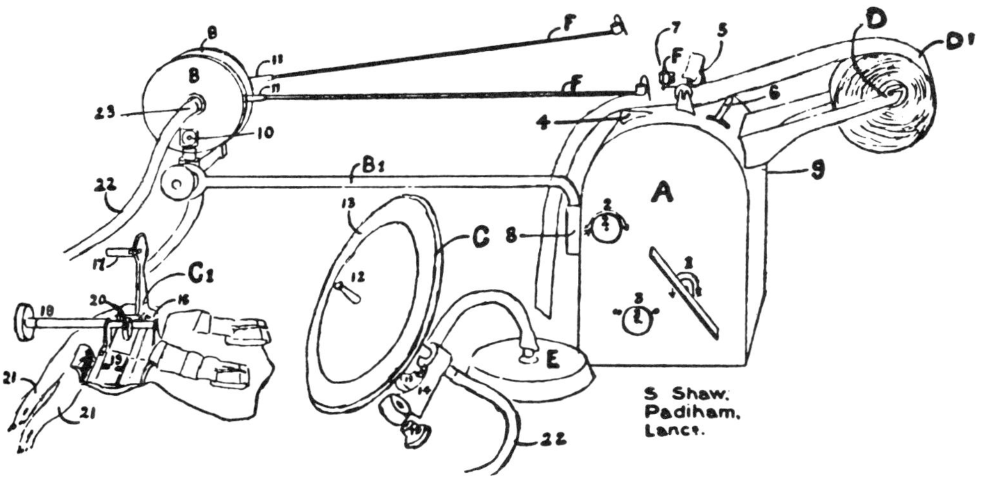

Fig. 6

James Mackenzie's Ink Polygraph. Hawkesley & Sons, Ltd. London: Catalogue. Not dated.

The complete outfit includes a clockwork motor with variable speeds, and a time-marker registering 1/5 seconds, two writing tambours, radial, jugular and cardiac receivers. There are two extra pens and one dozen rolls of paper.

virtues and faults, though it had been in use for fifteen years at this date. Other modern methods such as trichlorethylene, defibrillators and artificial circulation are not even mentioned. Nor is refrigeration anæsthesia, though this had been introduced six years earlier.[5]

The next book, published in the same year, 1948, is British, by Sir Thomas Lewis.[6] Sir Thomas was more or less Mackenzie's successor in cardiology, which now returned to the fold as the exclusive property of men working in hospitals and laboratories, after the surprising intrusion of a great general practitioner. He gives three and half pages out of 293 to anæsthesia and operations. The only anæsthetics mentioned at all are those which were all in use 48 years earlier—in 1900—chloroform, ether, nitrous oxide and spinals. One presumes that these represent the author's recollections of the days when he gave a few anæsthetics as a student. (He took his B.Sc. in 1902 and his M.D. in 1907, so the presumption is probably correct.) All newer developments—and there were plenty by

1948—are ignored completely. Cyclopropane and the intravenous barbiturates, which had been in use for fifteen years, are not mentioned, nor is ethylene, which is ten years older still; nor are relaxants and other recent methods, including helium, which might have rated a mention in a book dealing largely with dyspnoeic patients. Even local anæsthesia finds no mention, except for dental extractions. Status lymphaticus does not appear at all.

The next year another British book, of modest size this time,[7] failed to mention anæsthesia or the lymphatic state in its 256 pages.

In 1950 Paul Wood[8] could find no room, in 545 pages, to mention anæsthesia, except for two brief references to the mere fact that chloroform can cause ventricular fibrillation. There is a paragraph on death from sudden trauma:

> "Two factors seem important in these instances; a certain diathesis which used to be called status lymphaticus, but which is probably more related to suprarenal function; and a ventricle prone to fibrillation, as in elderly subjects, or in those with sub-clinical coronary artery disease."

The only comment which a historian can make upon this statement is that deaths attributed to status lymphaticus were almost invariably in young subjects. The condition was reported so frequently that unfortunately I did not make a note of every case. Of 9 deaths of which I have records, 6 were under anæsthesia. Of these 9 one may be excluded. He was a case of submucous resection of the septum. Adrenalin was injected locally and light chloroform anæsthesia was superimposed, so he was probably a case of primary heart failure due to ventricular fibrillation, who would have died in any case from this toxic combination. Of the remaining 8 the oldest was twenty-one and the next oldest fifteen and a half. These can hardly be called elderly, nor yet likely subjects for coronary disease, whether sub-clinical or not.

Of books on heart disease published in 1951 I examined three. The first[9] was American and contained 525 pages. Status lymphaticus does not appear, and anæsthesia only just. One paragraph of twelve lines is thought sufficient. The help which the anæsthetist may get from it may be judged by: "The choice (of anæsthetic) must remain an individual matter." This is just about as helpful as the famous definition of an archdeacon as one who performs archidiaconal functions. The only definite statement to which the author commits himself is that "ether is tolerated very well."

Paul White's book,[10] also American, is a massive volume of 963 pages. Two of them are about anæsthesia.

"Thymic disease. Hypertrophy or persistence of the thymus gland is not attended by heart disease, but is accompanied by general arterial hypoplasia. The cause of the sudden death in the so-called status lymphaticus and its reputed relationship to the thymus gland are still unsolved mysteries."

The third American book of this date[11] gives four and a half pages out of 633—a higher percentage than many of the others. Newer methods are at least mentioned, and a good bibliography on the subject is given on p. 630. Status lymphaticus is not mentioned.

William Evans,[12] a British author, gives two pages out of 542. As far as it goes the article is quite good. Thiopentone, hypothermia and defibrillators are at least mentioned, though status lymphaticus is not.

Diseases of the Heart, by Charles K. Friedberg,[13] is by far the best of the lot, so far as our special subject is concerned. This enormous book of 1,122 pages actually allots fifteen and a half pages to it, very nearly as much as all the other 11 books put together. All modern methods are discussed briefly, including cross-circulation techniques, cardiac by-passes, defibrillators, hypothermia and mechanical pump-oxygenators. Status lymphaticus is described shortly, with the comment that "the whole concept has been rejected."

The last volume, in what I suppose is a fairly representative selection from twentieth century books on the heart, is the most recent.[14] It is small, 218 pages, and compact, so compact that our subject is not mentioned at all.

Technically speaking, this chapter strays, as far as books consulted are concerned, outside my self-imposed limits of the first hundred years of anæsthesia. But it interested me, and had to be written. And in fairness to the cardiologists, I had to see if any of the more modern books had managed to progress beyond nineteenth century anæsthesia. On the whole they had not. No less than nine out of twelve text-books were obsolete when they were published, as far as our subject is concerned.

Is it any wonder, then, that I ask for some anæsthetist to be trained in cardiology? I cannot think that a subject of this importance and complexity is worthy of being dismissed in a few lines, or of being discussed in a couple of pages. Most of the authors' knowledge of anæsthesia, as revealed in these books, seems to be either limited or obsolete or both, and bounded by the little they learnt when students.

I am not arguing that new methods are necessarily better than old ones—that does not follow at all. They may be, or they may not, but so long as they exist and so long as they are used, their safety and utility should be evaluated as exactly as possible. That applies to both new and old methods alike. The one essential is that they should *not* be evaluated and recommended by people who know nothing, and care less, about anæsthesia.

References

[1] J. Lister (1883). Anaesthesia. In T. Holmes and J. W. Hulke, *A System of Surgery*, 3rd. ed. Part III.

[2] Sir James Mackenzie (1916). *Principles of Diagnosis and Treatment in Heart Affections.* London: Oxford University Press.

[3] Crighton Bramwell and John T. King (1942). *The Principles and Practice of Cardiology.* London: Oxford University Press.

[4] Aldo A. Luisada (1948). *Heart.* Baltimore: The Williams & Wilkins Company.

[5] Crossman, Allen, Hurley, Ruggiero and Warden (1942). *Curr. Res. Anesth.* Vol. 21. 245.

[6] Sir Thomas Lewis (1948). *Diseases of the Heart.* 4th ed. London: Macmillan.

[7] Geoffrey Bourne (1949). *An Introduction to Cardiology.* London: Arnold.

[8] Paul Wood (1950). *Diseases of the Heart and Circulation.* London: Eyre & Spottiswoode.

[9] Samuel A. Levine (1951). *Clinical Heart Disease.* 4th ed. Philadelphia: Saunders.

[10] Paul Dudley White (1951). *Heart Disease.* 4th ed. New York: Macmillan.

[11] Emanuel Goldberger (1951). *Heart Disease.* London: Kimpton.

[12] William Evans (1956). *Cardiology.* 2nd ed. London: Butterworth.

[13] Charles K. Friedberg (1956). *Diseases of the Heart.* 2nd ed. Philadelphia: Saunders.

[14] Crighton Bramwell (1959). *A Clinical Introduction to Heart Disease.* London: Oxford University Press.

CHAPTER 5

NATURAL ANÆSTHESIA

It is the merest commonplace to say that some people are less sensitive to pain than others—any doctor who has been in practice for more than a week will know that. It is even possible that in very rare and most exceptional cases the normal stoicism of the more equable individuals may be exaggerated into an ability to bear severe pain without flinching, quite apart from the well known cases of religious fervour which produce the same effect.

In fact there is such a case on record—but only one so far as I know. Paul F. Eve, Professor of Surgery in the Medical College of Georgia, reported it in 1849.[1] It was a Mr. A., who died at the age of fifty-six.

"So universal has been the application of the Divine curse to man, that, *to suffer* and *to live* are not only inseparable, but may be considered as synonymous terms. In the observation of more than twenty-three years, I have met with but a single exception to this apparently absolute law of our existence. . . .

"During a political campaign, not liking the appearance of a finger injured in an encounter, he bit it off himself and spat it upon the ground.

"He had at one time an ulcer on a toe, extending finally to the foot, which resisted treatment for nearly three years. Mr. A. told his physician at the time, and has since repeated the same statement, that from first to last, it never gave him the slightest pain.

"An abscess also formed in his hand, involving in its progress the whole fore-arm and arm, which became enormously swollen up to the body, and threated his life. The lancet had repeatedly and freely to be used, and was followed by a copious discharge of pus for several weeks. During the whole treatment he says he experienced no pain.

"He says he felt no pain when his eyes were operated upon for cataract. . . . I can vouch for his statue-like immovability during the second operation.

"When his neck was pustulated by tartar emetic ointment, he did not feel it, but ordered the application to be repeated.

"I made three incisions with a bistoury in his neck to relieve erysipelatous inflammation. He was so unconscious of the operation, that after it was performed he asked me to do it, that he might turn over on his back in bed. . . .

"It is proper to say that Mr. A. was a man of great probity, and never boasted of being insensible to pain. The only cause suggested for this truly

THE

QUESTION CONSIDERED;

IS IT JUSTIFIABLE TO ADMINISTER CHLOROFORM IN SURGICAL OPERATIONS, AFTER ITS HAVING ALREADY PROVED SUDDENLY FATAL IN UPWARDS OF FIFTY CASES, WHEN PAIN CAN BE SAFELY PREVENTED, WITHOUT LOSS OF CONSCIOUSNESS, BY MOMENTARY BENUMBING COLD?

BY

JAMES ARNOTT, M.D.,

LATE SUPERINTENDENT OF THE MEDICAL ESTABLISHMENT AT ST. HELENA.

LONDON:
JOHN CHURCHILL, PRINCES STREET, SOHO.

1854.

FIG. 7

Mr. James Arnott's booklet. Despite his verbose and long-winded title, he is very definite in his preferences. He mentions the case of Hannah Greener, and also that of John Shorter, at St. Thomas's Hospital, who also died suddenly on October 10, 1849, while having a toe-nail removed—an identical and equally trivial operation. John Snow's list of chloroform deaths includes 36 cases up to the end of 1853 and 43 up to the end of 1854. Mr. Arnott must have discovered a few extra deaths, as he refers to "upwards of fifty cases"; there was certainly some reason for his fear of chloroform and his desire to replace it by something less dangerous.

PAINLESS TOOTH-EXTRACTION

WITHOUT CHLOROFORM.

WITH

OBSERVATIONS ON

LOCAL ANÆSTHESIA BY CONGELATION

IN

GENERAL SURGERY.

BY

WALTER BLUNDELL.

SURGEON-DENTIST.

LONDON:

JOHN CHURCHILL, NEW BURLINGTON STREET,

MDCCCLIV.

FIG. 8

The dentists also took up freezing or "congelation" as a substitute for chloroform. Mr. Blundell, also in 1854, stated that James Arnott had introduced the method in 1848. He claims that the wound heals better, that 75% of all operations can be done with it, and that the use of chloroform in dentistry is not justifiable.

DENTAL ANÆSTHESIA.

PAINLESS TOOTH EXTRACTION

BY

CONGELATION.

BY

J. RICHARD QUINTON.

Fourth Edition, Enlarged.

LONDON:

R. THEOBALD, 26, PATERNOSTER ROW.

MDCCCLVI.

FIG. 9

Mr. Richard Quinton, two years later, also wrote on the subject. By this time, according to Snow's list, there had been 47 deaths. Quinton stressed the importance of relieving pain, but held that general anæsthesia was too risky for dental operations. By general anæsthesia, of course, he meant chloroform. He stated that gradual freezing was not at all painful. This pamphlet was obviously written for the lay public as a sort of advertisement. It is long and verbose, but the method actually used is never described, and the booklet is useless to any dentist wishing to try the method.

singular and peculiar condition . . . is the free use of alcoholic potations. . . . But others have drunk more than he ever did, without producing the same result."

This is quite a different thing from the big game hunters' experiences which are recorded below. It is even more rare, it covers pain only and probably not the complete absence of fear that they felt as well. Also this was permanent, whereas theirs was a temporary condition, covering the time of crisis and no more.

There are other varieties of more or less natural anæsthesia, which are easier to understand. Baron Larrey performed many painless operations on half-frozen soldiers during the intense cold of the Russian winter which defeated Napoleon. For this reason—because he had seen with his own eyes that painless surgery was just possible in exceptional circumstances—he was the only man who was open-minded enough to be interested in Hickman's claims to have produced anæsthesia by the inhalation of carbon dioxide.

In the very early days of inhalation anæsthesia the number of deaths from chloroform caused much alarm. Dr. James Arnott was very worried about them which made him an enthusiastic upholder of what he called congelation, or freezing with a mixture of ice and salt.[2] He claimed that it was perfectly safe, which chloroform was not, that it never failed when properly employed, that it could be used in all external operations, and for the first stage of amputations. It was not painful, he stated, if the freezing and the thawing were done gradually. He admitted that it took a little longer to act in the presence of inflammation; but it was beneficial in that it prevented erysipelas. He also tried to prove that the mortality of amputations in London hospitals had increased by 12 per cent. since the pre-chloroform days, but his figures would not convince a modern statistician.

Ice and salt was a little inconvenient to handle and difficult to control in spite of Dr. Arnott's enthusiasm, and Benjamin Ward Richardson designed[3] a more convenient way of achieving the same result by freezing. His ether spray could be applied more exactly to the required spot, and an attempt could even be made to freeze the deeper structures in stages, in advance of the knife, and so obtain more efficient anæsthesia in amputations than was possible with the old ice-and-salt bags.

After this, of course, the ether spray was itself replaced by the still more convenient ethyl chloride tube, which required no pumping. This continued to hold a small place in anæsthesia for little incisions in restricted areas.

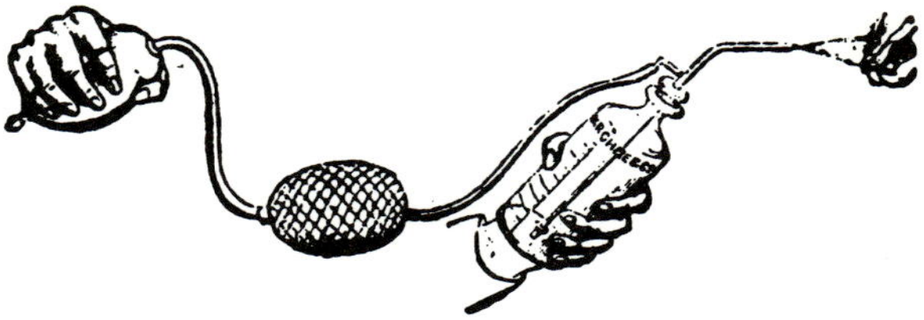

FIG. 10

Medical Times and Gazette. 1866, Feb. 3. 116. Benjamin Ward Richardson.
Ether spray for local anæsthesia by freezing. 5 column article.

In 1942 Arnott's congelation was revived under the name of refrigeration anæsthesia.[4] A thirteen page article described its use for major surgery on the limbs, such as amputations for gangrene.

Other methods of more or less natural anæsthesia have been tried. Benjamin Lee,[5] in 1880, told how a patient went to Dr. Bonwill, a dentist in Philadelphia. He made her breathe as fast as she could for several minutes and took out the tooth without pain. Dr. Lee speculates whether this was a form of hypnotism, or whether it was due to a modification of the cerebral circulation brought about by the rapid breathing. Dr. Bonwill had used the method for years. The breathing must be really rapid—at least 100 per minute. He thought it was partly due to diversion of the attention, partly to lack of carbon dioxide and partly to slowing of the blood flow causing hyperaemia of the brain.

Two years later, in 1882, W. A. Berridge reported successful use of the rapid breathing method.[6] He had reduced two dislocations and a strangulated hernia with its aid. He pointed out that the doctor must show the patient how to do it and encourage him to breathe hard, breathe deeply and breathe faster and faster. Half measures were no use at all.

Dr. L. Steiner of Sourabaya described[7] a method of anæsthesia used by the natives of Java. It consisted of pressure on the neck until the patient was unconscious. He considered that it was due to compression of the carotids. The fact that there was no change in the pulse or the pupil indicated that pressure on the vagus or sympathetic was not the cause.

Dr. Neil Macleod, in 1886,[8] reported a method of reducing dislocations of the shoulder without pain. He had only tried it in 2 cases, but claimed success in both. As an aid to relaxation the patient was lying down. Then instead of a straight pull with a foot in the axilla he pulled with the arm at right angles to the trunk. He said that this gave much better relaxation and much less pain.

It is doubtful whether the next case should really appear in this chapter at all, because a drug, a very familiar drug, was in fact used. In 1852, when people were beginning to fear chloroform for its treachery, a man of twenty-two was caught by the revolving shaft of a steam engine.[9] His right leg was torn off at the knee joint, and above this level there was a fracture of the femur. The left knee joint was laid open and the femur on that side dislocated. There was nothing for it but amputation through both thighs.

It was in fact a bad-risk case which would have made a modern anæsthetist choose his anæsthetic and his method very carefully, after using to their full extent all the up-to-date devices for resuscitation. But in those days there was practically no choice. Ether and nitrous oxide had both dropped out of use, killed by the initial triumphs of chloroform, and were not resurrected until many years later. Oxygen was practically never available, because it had to be manufactured on the spot, and transfusions were not only rare but risky in those days. Neither asepsis nor blood groups were known, so any blood transfused was certainly dirty and very probably incompatible as well. In practice therefore the choice was either chloroform—or not. Perhaps wisely, the surgeon chose to operate without anæsthesia. But not without pre-medication, for the patient had a pint of brandy during the three hours before the operation—an English pint of 20 ounces, not an American pint of 16 ounces. He also took brandy almost continuously during the operation.

How efficient this unorthodox but powerful pre-medication was in preventing pain is not recorded—but it should have been fairly effective. Anyway the patient recovered. But what an appalling hangover he must have had!

The problem of pain has been a long-established stumbling-block for philosophers. The late C. E. M. Joad was very much worried by it, and had great difficulty in reconciling it with belief in a beneficient Deity, though he finally did so.

It is rather a pity that the average philosopher has had no medical training. As he takes the whole of knowledge for his province he tends to be somewhat scornful of its branches. But he misses something by this attitude. He cannot visualise, for example, a case of Morvan's disease. He has almost certainly never heard of it, though it is a complaint which ought to fulfil the philosopher's ideal. The patient has large areas of his body devoid of all feeling, so that pain, at any rate in these areas, simply does not exist. The result is, of course, that the patient becomes a mass of cuts, burns, bruises and other injuries of all kinds. It is not even safe for him to smoke a cigarette, lest he burn his fingers to the bone without knowing it.

Nor does the philosopher take note of a trivial medical incident which happens tens of thousands of times a year. It is especially common in engineering works, but may happen to anybody anywhere. Foreign bodies in the eye are very frequent and very uncomfortable—so uncomfortable that their possessors lose no time in having them removed as soon as possible—painlessly, thanks to Karl Koller and his cocaine. What the armchair critics forget is the fact that, if the cornea was not very sensitive to pain, the fragments of road-dust or metal would be allowed to remain until the eye was irrevocably damaged. They also do not realise that vast numbers of women discover a lump in the breast and ignore it until it is too late, merely because it is not painful. If only carcinoma was painful in its early stages the surgeon would operate upon a much larger percentage of curable cases.

Even the annual reports of the Medical Defence Unions would make instructive reading for the armchair thinkers. Not many years go by without some surgeon being sued for heavy damages because somebody has left an uncovered hot water bottle in bed with a patient who is just back from the theatre after an operation. By the time the patient recovers consciousness he has a severe burn which costs somebody a considerable amount per square inch.

But our imaginary philosopher may shift his ground at this stage. He will perhaps admit by now that some pain can be useful and indeed protective. But he will still point to the unnecessary cruelty and pain which is a result of that stern law—eat or be eaten. Watch a domestic cat, which may be a devoted mother and a gentle pet, playing with a half-dead mouse with a terrible sadistic joy. Here is cruelty for its own sake—as pointless as the mediaeval torture chamber and as hideously useless as the Gestapo. The only reply to this is another question—does the mouse really suffer? Are you sure?

This makes the philosopher indignant. Are you arguing that the mouse—a living, sentient animal—feels no pain? That it feels no terror or despair at its hopeless situation? The philosopher naturally assumes that the mouse can feel fear and pain much the same as a human being feels them. This must be his theory, for if he thought mice had no more

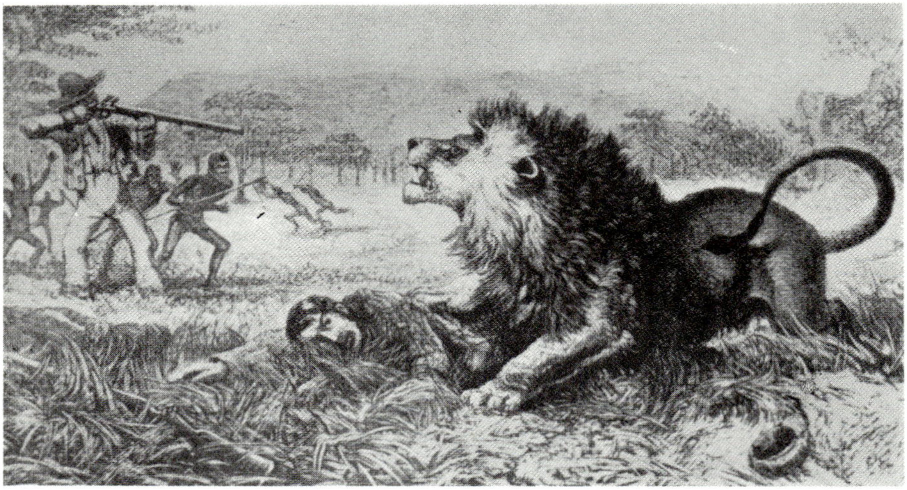

PLATE XX

Livingstone and the lion. From *Missionary Travels and Researches in South Africa.* David Livingstone, M.D. 1875 Plate opposite page 1. London: John Murray.

The flintlock gun aimed by the valiant Mebalwe missed fire at this critical moment! The artist appears to have provided him with one barrel only; it was, as a matter of fact, a double-barrelled gun, but as both of them missed fire, it didn't help much. Mebalwe was the next one to be attacked.

feeling than stones or lumps of coal he would not be bothering about them at all. The problem of pain would not arise.

Let me say at once that I agree entirely with this merciful hypothesis. I think a mouse can feel the prick of a pin just as a man does. But instead of guessing we ought to collect some definite evidence as to what really is felt by a mouse in a perfectly hopeless position. This is not so impossible as it sounds. Plenty of human mice have been in the same situation, for remember that there are very large cats as well as small ones. These humans, who are quite certainly capable of feeling fear, pain, terror and panic, because they can describe their sensations to us, may not, and very often do not, feel anything of the sort in a similar situation.

My first witness is David Livingstone, the famous Scottish medical missionary, who was born in 1813. He spent sixteen years in Africa at a time when the interior of the continent was almost unknown, from 1840 to 1856. In 1843 lions were a great nuisance in the village of Mabotsa—but he shall tell the story in his own words:[10]

"They (the tribe) went once to attack the animals, but, being rather cowardly in comparison with the Bechuanas in general, they returned without slaying any. It is well known that if one in a troop of lions is killed the remainder leave that part of the country. The next time, therefore, the herds were attacked, I went with the people to encourage them to rid themselves of the annoyance by destroying one of the marauders. We found the animals on a small hill covered with trees. The men formed round it in a circle, and gradually closed up as they advanced. (I was) below on the plain with a native schoolmaster named Mebalwe. . . . In going round the end of the hill I saw a lion sitting on a piece of rock, about thirty yards off, with a little bush in front of him. I took a good aim at him through the bush, and fired both barrels into it. The men called out, 'He is shot, he is shot! . . . let us go to him!' I saw the lion's tail erected in anger, and turning to the people, said, 'Stop a little till I load again'. When in the act of ramming down the bullets I heard a shout, and, looking half round, I saw the lion in the act of springing upon me."

Loading a muzzle loader was a slow process in those days, very unlike slipping another cartridge or two into a modern rifle or gun. The correct amount of powder had to be tipped down the barrel from a powder flask, then a wad had to be pushed down with the ramrod, then the bullet dropped in and another wad rammed down to prevent it falling out. Then the cap had to be put on in a percussion gun or the priming pan filled with powder in a flint gun. It was a matter of minutes rather than seconds, as now.

"He caught me by the shoulder, and we both came to the ground together. Growling horribly, he shook me as a terrier dog does a rat. The shock produced a stupor similar to that which seems to be felt by a mouse after the first gripe of the cat. It caused a sort of dreaminess, in which there was no sense of pain nor feeling of terror, though I was quite conscious of all that was happening. It was like what patients partially under the influence of chloroform describe; they see the operation, but do not feel the knife."

This remark confirms much evidence from other sources that anæsthesia, at that time, was almost always very light indeed.

"This placidity is probably produced in all animals killed by the carnivora; and if so, is a merciful provision of the Creator for lessening the pain of death. As he had one paw on the back of my head, I turned round to relieve myself of the weight, and saw his eyes directed to Mebalwe, who was aiming at him from a distance of ten to fifteen yards. His gun, which was a flint one, missed fire in both barrels."

Liability to misfire was one of the weak points of the flint lock, especially in its cheaper forms. Although the more reliable and rainproof percussion cap had been in use for over twenty years, flint locks were still in use in the British Army until 1842, the year before this incident. So they would be universal in cheap trade-guns made for export to natives. Many are still in use, for flint-knappers, who belong to one of the oldest trades in the world, still produce gun flints.

"The animal immediately left me to attack him, and bit his thigh. Another man, whose life I had saved after he had been tossed by a buffalo, attempted to spear the lion, upon which he turned from Mebalwe and seized this fresh foe by the shoulder. At that moment the bullets the beast had received took effect, and he fell down dead. The whole was the work of a few moments, and must have been his paroxysm of dying rage. . . . Besides crunching the bone into splinters, eleven of his teeth had penetrated the upper part of my arm. The bite of a lion resembles a gunshot wound. It is generally followed by a great deal of sloughing and discharge, and ever afterwards pains are felt periodically in the part. I had on a tartan jacket, which I believe wiped off the virus from the teeth that pierced the flesh, for my two companions in the affray have both suffered from the normal pains, while I escaped with only the inconvenience of a false joint in my limb."

When Livingstone died on May 1st, 1873, his body was carried back to civilisation by his native servants and friends. It was identified by this ununited fracture of the humerus.

David Livingstone was brought up the hard way. He went to work in a factory in 1823, when he was ten years old. With his first week's wages he bought a book *Rudiments of Latin*. His working hours were from 6 a.m. to 8 p.m.—fourteen hours. Then he went to evening school from 8 to 10 p.m. and continued work at home until midnight. At the age of nineteen he became a cotton spinner and somehow managed to support himself as a medical student, for he had conceived the idea of serving his fellow men as a medical missionary. He went to Africa in 1840, the voyage to the Cape taking three months.

Was this the sort of man to lie about his encounter with the lion? Is it likely, with his strong religious beliefs? What would be the object of lying, anyway? No, if human testimony is ever to be believed at all, this story must be accepted as the literal truth. To suspect Livingstone of lying is to my mind far more difficult than to believe his story.

And, this is not a solitary instance, a mere *lusus naturae*. Sir Lyon Playfair[11] quotes, not only this case but two others.

"I have known three friends who were partially devoured by wild beasts, under apparently hopeless circumstances. . . . The first was Livingstone. . . . He assured me that he felt no fear or pain, and that his only feeling was one of intense curiosity as to which part of his body the lion would take next."

This almost amusing comment is omitted from Livingstone's own account, but fits in well with the similar thoughts of the Turkish Ambassador.

"The next was Rustem Pasha, now Turkish Ambassador in London. A bear attacked him and tore off part of his hand and part of his arm and shoulder. He also assured me that he had neither pain nor fear, but that he felt excessively angry because the bear grunted with so much satisfaction in munching him. The third case is that of Sir Edward Bradford, an Indian officer, now occupying a high position in the India Office."

Sir Edward Ridley Colborne Bradford (1836-1911) later became Commissioner of the Metropolitation Police. The accident occurred on 10th May, 1863.

"He was seized by a tiger . . . which deliberately devoured the whole of his arm, beginning at the hand and ending at the shoulder. He was positive that he had no sensation of fear, and thinks that he felt a little pain when the fangs went through his hand, but is certain that he felt none during the munching of his arm."

Again, John Taylor, a famous big-game shot, who was a professional elephant hunter for twenty-five years[12] and who wrote a book on big-game rifles,[13] had a similar experience.

"(*Pondoro,* p. 22). His (the leopard's) face was only about two or three feet from mine when I saw him; he was actually in the air and coming down. I just had time to draw my revolver and shoot him in the chest when he landed on top of me. His weight brought me down and the back of my head made contact with a stone or something which scattered my wits. I can just dimly remember moving my head slightly to one side so that he would not chew my ear off, as his jaws were clashing immediately beside it. I could feel his claws busy on chest and thigh, but curiously felt no pain. Then there came a splintering crack and thump: Joro, hearing the report of the revolver, had brought the butt of the rifle down with a crash on the leopard's head. It was an extremely plucky thing to do. . . . His blow smashed the butt off the rifle, but it put a stop to the leopard's antics—which was maybe just as well, because all the ribs down the right side of my chest were exposed and my left thigh was in ribbons.

(p. 24). "I have described this incident in some detail because I have heard so many discussions as to the amount of pain a man must suffer when being mauled by a beast. Apart from my own experience I know personally some seven or eight others who have been mauled by lion, tiger or leopard, in addition to the many others I have heard or read about, and they all say the same thing: that they felt no pain at all during the actual mauling. I myself had a curious detached feeling, quite impersonal, as though I were withdrawn and watching the predicament in which some other fellow found himself. (It was exactly the same years later, under a wounded and very angry elephant). It is true that I was somewhat dazed by the leopard's sudden attack. However, I was quite conscious and could definitely feel his claws busy. But there was no pain."

This evidence confirms Livingstone's experience exactly—if any confirmation were necessary. But even more extraordinary than the absence of pain in this case is the amazing speed of an expert's reactions. The leopard sprang from a tree, and his first sight of it was when it was in the air about a yard away—and yet he had time, not only to draw his revolver but to fire it. This incredibly quick reaction makes the television cowboys look like slow-motion paralytics.

During and after the war I asked many men whether they felt pain at the moment when they were wounded. As far as I remember, not one of them did, however badly they were injured. The pain came on later, of course. We must conclude, therefore, that natural anæsthesia exists, whether we explain it by nervous shock, by self-hypnosis, or whether we accept Livingstone's simple explanation that it is a merciful provision of the Creator.

After Nan had read the typescript of this essay she produced one of her usual sensible suggestions. "Circuses," she said: "why don't you get some more evidence from lion-tamers who have been mauled?"

The first large circus did not reply to my letter—one of the very few times I found any correspondent unhelpful. The second one was unable to help, so thus far I have no extra evidence to bring forward.

References

[1] Paul F. Eve (1849). *Sth. med. surg. J.* Vol. 5, N.S. 718.
[2] *Med. Times and Gaz.* (1857), Feb. 7. 135.
[3] *Med. Times and Gaz.* (1866), Feb. 3. 116.
[4] Lyman Weeks Crossman, Frederick W. Allen, Vincent Hurley, Wilfred Ruggiero and Cyrus E. Warden (1942). *Curr. Res. Anesth.* Vol. 21. 241.
[5] *Brit. med. J.* (1880), Oct. 16. 628.
[6] *Brit. med. J.* (1882), Nov. 25. 1038.
[7] *Brit. med. J.* (1902), July 26. 270.
[8] *Brit. med. J.* (1886), Jan. 30. 194.
[9] *Brit. med. J.* (1852), July 21. 363.
[10] David Livingstone (1875). *A Popular Account of Missionary Travels and Researches in South Africa,* p. 10. London: Murray.
[11] *Brit. med. J.* (1889), Mar. 2. 489.
[12] John Taylor (1956). *Pondoro. Last of the Ivory Hunters.* London: Muller.
[13] John Taylor (1948). *Big Game and Big Game Rifles.* London: Jenkins.

CHAPTER 6

LATENT PERIODS

"Wonderful little, when all is said,
Wonderful little our fathers knew.
Half of their remedies cured you dead—
Most of their teaching was quite untrue—"

—RUDYARD KIPLING.

THE time lag of many discoveries and new ideas is incredibly long. For instance, Humphry Davy (1778-1829) suggested the use of nitrous oxide in surgery in 1800, a suggestion which was repeated when the book was reprinted in his collected works in 1839. Forty-six years went by before Wells first tried it.

Professor Schroff noted the numbing effect of cocaine on the tongue in 1862, after Albert Niemann had isolated the alkaloid in 1859, but this observation waited for twenty-two years before Karl Koller (1857-1944) put it into practical use in ophthalmology in 1884.

Chloroform was discovered independently by three different chemists in 1831, but it was not used as an anæsthetic until sixteen years later. Ether was the most neglected of all anæsthetic agents. It waited patiently for 306 years from the time of Valerius Cordus to Morton—or 302 if one counts C. W. Long's incredibly secretive trials in Jefferson, Georgia.

Latent periods of new ideas are not confined to anæsthesia by any means. They occur in all branches of knowledge. Leeuwenhoek first saw bacteria under the microscope two hundred years before Pasteur put forward his theory that they might cause disease. Oliver Wendell Holmes (1809-1897) very nearly penetrated the secret of puerperal sepsis in 1843, Ignaz Phillip Semmelweiss did the same, quite independently in 1847, and both of them produced remarkable results. Semmelweiss cut the mortality rate of hospital midwifery cases from 12 per cent. to 3 per cent. in six months. Another account states that before his time the mortality of the Vienna Lying-in Hospital, from 1840 to 1846, had the appalling mortality of 2,260 deaths in 22,120 confinements, a death rate of 1 in 10, which was reduced to 1 in 74 by cleaner midwifery.

But neither of them could make any headway against the god-of-things-as-they-are, and they met with violent opposition. Holmes discreetly retired from medicine altogether and devoted himself to the less dangerous and less frustrating atmosphere of poetry and literature.

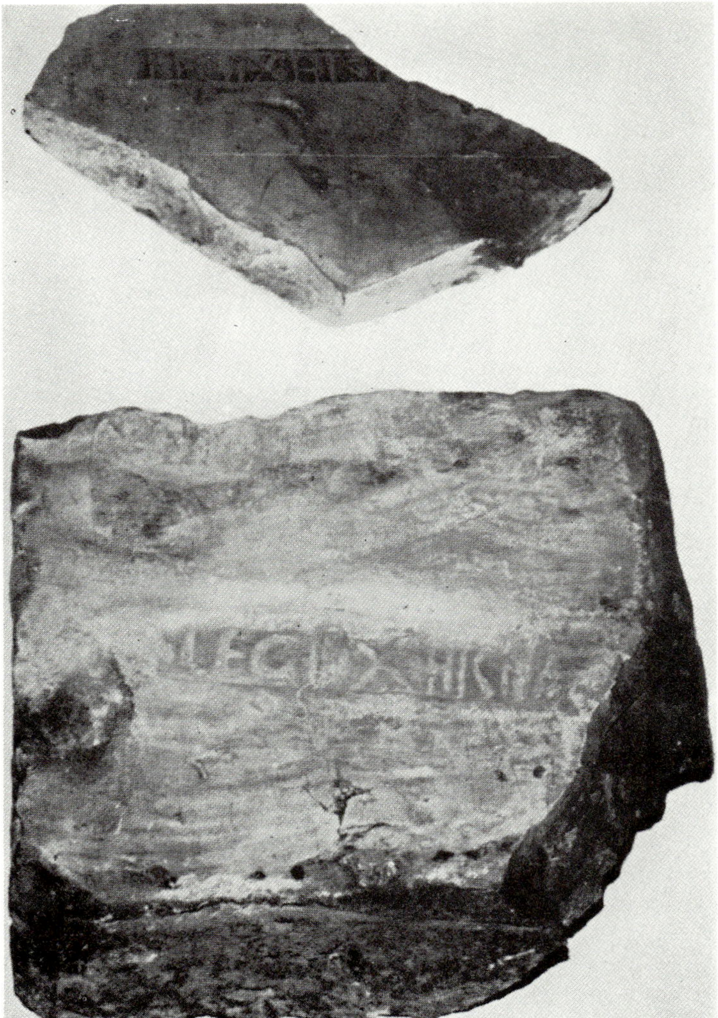

PLATE XXI

Legend on page 81

Semmelweiss fought on valiantly, but finally became insane and, ironically enough, died from the very septicæmia which he had done so much to prevent. Twenty-four years after Holmes' pioneer attempt and twenty years after Semmelweiss's valuable but underrated work, Lister (in 1867) drew aside the veil of dirt from surgery and prevailed upon his colleagues to accept his methods. Slowly and reluctantly they did this —his results forced them, or some of them, into it. Those whose prejudice could not be shaken even by facts were in due course—mercifully for their patients—removed by the hand of death.

More incredible still, Hero of Alexandria designed the first jet engine in the first century A.D. It was only a toy, so simple that it is difficult to decide whether it should be called a turbine or a jet, but it waited nearly two thousand years before use was made of it. Parsons developed his first turbine in 1884 and Heinkel made a jet aeroplane which made its first flight in Germany in 1939. Frank Whittle designed and made the first jet engine to fly in England in 1941.

This perhaps holds the record with the longest latent period of all. But there are others nearly as surprising. All over the Roman Empire the legions made roofing tiles for their barracks, which were stamped with the unit's name and number. Gaulish manufacturers who made the red Samian pottery for table and domestic use at the same period of history all stamped their name or trademark on their wares. Both these

PLATE XXI

"All over the Roman Empire the legions made roofing tiles for their barracks, which were stamped with the unit's name and number."

These two are stamped LEG IX HIS, the mark of Legio IX, Hispana, the Spanish Legion, which took part in the invasion of Britain in A.D. 42. It was stationed at York, until it was overwhelmed and destroyed about 120 A.D. It disappeared from the Army List and was never re-formed. Its place as the York garrison was taken by Legio VI, Victrix.

The destruction of Legio IX, a mighty force of 6,000 disciplined swordsmen, was one of the utter disasters of history. It was on a much larger scale than the defeat of Custer and the 7th U.S. Cavalry at the Little Big Horn in 1876, when the General and his 226 men were all killed; or than the British disaster at Isandlwana three years later, when 800 men were attacked by 10,000 Zulus and all but 40 exterminated.

Photo taken by the author in York.

things were mass-produced and can be seen in their thousands in museums all over England and the Continent—continents, rather, for the Roman Empire overflowed into Asia and parts of Africa. But, until Gutenberg fifteen hundred years later, nobody thought of using stamps like these to print books.

Even when our well known drugs and methods had at last managed to force their way into use, it generally took a long time to discover their disadvantages. Simpson published his very short six-day experience of chloroform on November 10th, 1847. Its liability to cause sudden heart failure did not become potentially apparent until January 28th, 1848, when Hannah Greener died like a shot rabbit under the hands of Dr. Meggison—an interval of eleven weeks and two days. I say 'potentially apparent' because many different explanations were given to account for this tragedy—and for the stream of others which followed it. Simpson himself attributed the death to the methods of resuscitation which were employed. He quite frankly said that Hannah was drowned by the brandy and water which was poured into her mouth while she was unconscious. He was right about the dangers of this practice, but in this case it probably made no difference. Hannah was dead already, of that there is very little doubt.

Not unnaturally it took a long time before chloroform enthusiasts could be convinced of the truth of the seemingly impossible—that too small a dose could kill. They would willingly admit that too large a dose could be fatal, generally with the reservation—until they met with a death in their own practice—that this could only happen to other people and not to themselves. Their method was infallible—if only others could be induced to see it. Edward Lawrie was later one of the protagonists of this school, whose doctrines had been raised almost to the rank of theological dogma by Simpson, Syme and Lister. But the argument was—and it appeared to be absolutely watertight—that it was not possible to get drunk by drinking too little whisky.

Many never did become convinced that it could happen, in spite of the fact that it was constantly happening. Every week the journals reported sudden deaths under chloroform anæsthesia for trivial operations. But whole generations of users had died before Goodman Levy's classic experiments with adrenalin in light chloroform anæsthesia explained the mystery in 1911, no less than sixty-three years after Hannah Greener's death.[1, 2, 3]

The combination of light—not deep—chloroform anæsthesia and adrenalin produced fatal ventricular fibrillation experimentally. Fear produces excess of adrenalin in the blood. This explained everything. It explained why the fatalities were usually young, healthy people who were undergoing trivial operations only. The bad risk cases for serious operations concentrated their thoughts on the operation doing them good—it could hardly make them worse. It explained the immunity of women in labour from these sudden deaths, because they did not fear the anæsthetic but clamoured for it.

J. A. Bodine of New York[4] got very near to the truth on clinical evidence alone, but did not bring forward any experimental evidence in support of his theory. He pointed out the similarity of death from light chloroform anæsthesia and death from fright. He also mentioned the well known immunity of obstetric cases. He quoted one patient who died of fright before any chloroform had been given, and another who died from an enema which he thought was the first step of an operation for hæmorrhoids.

Much earlier Dr. Jeanell, a Frenchman, had had the same idea.[5] He thought the deaths were due to fright. He advised getting consent for the operation without fixing the day. Then a 'trial' is made to ascertain whether it is possible to cause sleep. The 'trial' is, of course, the actual anæsthetic itself. Dr. Jeanell was not only a precursor of Levy, but also of Crile and his anoci-association method. This was one of the few continental contributions of value to inhalation anæsthesia. It passed quite unnoticed at the time.

No date, of course, can be given for the discovery of the fact that death from overdosage could occur. This was axiomatic, self-evident from the beginning, and the reports of early anæsthetic cases convince one that it could rarely, if ever, have occurred at that time. The outstanding feature about all the early case records is that none of them was ever properly under. This can be deduced, among other things, from the induction times when these are given. Adult patients with no premedication whatever were constantly stated to be 'under' in a minute and a half or two minutes with ether or chloroform—not nitrous oxide, mark you, or any other quick acting drug. There is frequently other evidence to the effect that the patient moved or had to be held down during the operation. Surgeons who had learned their trade on conscious patients were well used to this, and it called for no comment. They were not fussy, and there was no elaborate aseptic ritual to be spoiled by a movement or two. Or patients were given drinks when 'under'. Sometimes they even replied to questions in a dreamy way. The *Lancet* (1847, Jan. 9. 54) reports an amputation through the thigh at Bristol

General Hospital. The operator was Mr. J. G. Lansdown. Ether was given from an inhaler designed by Mr. Herapath. It was stated to be successful and painless. The depth of the anæsthesia can be judged from the report, which states that wine was given at intervals during the operation. Not until the advent of abdominal surgery in the 1880s was deep anæsthesia with its accompanying immobility demanded or expected.

The third cause of chloroform deaths—delayed chloroform poisoning—did not attract attention until 1894, after the drug had been in use for forty-seven years, when L. G. Guthrie[6] described a series of 10 cases in children—9 of them fatal. Even then the chloroform enthusiasts would have none of it at first. When this rare but very fatal and completely unpreventable complication happened it was attributed to carbolic acid poisoning, sepsis, fat embolism—anything but the chloroform. The fact that it escaped notice for so long is not surprising. No detailed records of anæsthesia were kept in those days—it was not regarded as important. It was a simple easy job which could be relegated to anybody—or so surgeons thought. And the symptoms did not come on immediately, but after a delay of perhaps forty-eight hours, long after the other effects of the anæsthetic had apparently passed off. This meant that its connection with the anæsthetic was not obvious at first sight.

Status lymphaticus as a cause of death was recorded in 1860.[7] Paltauf wrote a paper on it in 1889,[8] and by 1907 it had become a very popular explanation of death during anæsthesia. Later, doubt was cast upon its very existence as a reality. The *Lancet* published a leading article in 1931 entitled "The end of status lymphaticus." Were the older school of pathologists right, or the newer ones? It is anybody's guess. What is certain is that they can't both be right. Sir Bernard Spilsbury, a pathologist of vast experience, whose evidence sent many murderers to the scaffold, certainly believed in it. So did the two John Glaisters, father and son.

Apart from a temporary eclipse of its popularity for two decades after the introduction of chloroform—and this was not universal, for many centres kept faithful to ether all the time—ether had been in world-wide use for eighty years and everything possible seemed to be known about it, when suddenly in 1926 an epidemic of ether convulsions appeared. There had been a few cases before, but only a few.[9, 10] The previous lack of reported cases could not be attributed, in this instance, to the absence of record-keeping which was certainly usual in those days and which was responsible for some of these conditions being missed.

Nobody could miss, or fail to observe, ether convulsions. Occurring as they did during actual anæsthesia, and deep anæsthesia at that, they were far too unprecedented, too dramatic, too dangerous and too obviously directly connected with the anæsthesia to be overlooked. If they had not been reported before it was because they had not occurred. It is easy to explain their absence in the early days, for the anæsthesia was always too light for them to happen. Ether tremor there may have been, but not convulsions. These could not possibly be mistaken for the transient and harmless tremor of light anæsthesia.

As long ago as 1930 I became interested in the subject, having had a fatal case myself. A search of the literature produced twelve different theories of their causation, many of them mutually contradictory and none of them fitting the facts. So I added a thirteenth theory of my own to the list.[11] This was probably just as fallacious as any of the others.*

Carbon dioxide absorption is usually attributed to Dennis Jackson and Ralph Waters, who certainly revived it and popularised it. But they were by no means the originators, for it has a respectably long history, which actually began many years before anæsthesia itself. Stephen Hales (1677-1761) tried it soon after 1700, and Johann Ingenhousz (1730-1799) experimented with it in 1782, both using lime water as their absorbent. The first mention of it in connection with anæsthesia is in 1868[12] when Ibbetson reported 3 cases of nitrous oxide given in a closed circuit by Mr. Coleman.

> "A quantity of the gas amounting to one-third of that usually required to produce anæsthesia was inhaled out of a small India rubber bag; and an apparatus was so arranged in connection with it that the products of exhalation from the lungs were passed over recently slacked lime, and then reconveyed into the same bag. By this arrangement the gas was inhaled over and over again, the hydrate of lime removing the carbonic acid gas given off by the lungs. The gas was in no way impaired in quality, producing anæsthesia as efficiently and in the same time as that which has been inhaled only once. The quantity in the small bag sufficed for two patients, affecting a saving therefore of about four-sixths."

About two months later Alfred Coleman himself reported more than 100 cases done by this method.[13] The agent used was quicklime, recently and only partially slaked. They were all successful, except 3 cases, occurring in succession, where much excitement took place. The lime was found to be saturated with water and carbon dioxide.

*The number of theories has now risen to 32.

Just over a year afterwards Richard Rendle[14] reported 24 cases using Coleman's method. He took the precaution of leaving the expiratory valve open for the first three breaths in order to get rid of the residual air in the lungs, an extremely sensible thing to do when using this method.

Jackson's first absorption machine was brought out in 1915—one hundred and thirty three years later than Ingenhousz's and forty-seven years after Coleman's. Closed circuit absorption, using soda-lime and the Waters' canister, was in full swing at Madison, Wisconsin, in 1933, when I visited there, and cyclopropane was being extensively tried out as a very new anæsthetic. This gas, of course, made the method virtually essential on the grounds of economy. It was far too expensive to be allowed to run to waste out of an expiratory valve merely because some excess carbon dioxide had to be let out as well. So the increasing employment of cyclopropane meant that the closed circuit became very popular. Its use soon spread to other anæsthetics, mainly nitrous oxide and ether, and within these limits it was both safe and satisfactory.

But in 1944 two reports were published[15] of a new and unprecedented complication. Disastrous nerve palsies were found to follow trichlorethylene anæsthesia when, and only when, it was used in conjunction with soda-lime. It was found that the two substances caused a chemical reaction to take place, with the production of dichloroacetylene. In the first paper 13 cases were recorded, accompanied by herpes in 9 of them. There were 2 deaths in this series. Moreover, once trichlorethylene had contaminated the soda-lime, toxic effects could be produced by the use of the same canister in other cases, even those in which no trichlorethylene had been used.

Ordinary explosions due to open fires, gas jets and lighted candles, hazards which were much commoner in Victorian age operating rooms than they are now, must have been noticed from the very early days. Charles Thomas Jackson, Morton's phony competitor for the honour of first using ether, foresaw this danger when he advised the use of a safety lamp in operations about the mouth and face. W. Channing[16] also foresaw this danger, and in one case covered the sponge with paper. Another suggestion was to use a piece of bladder as a mask cover, but Dr. Hayward said that this might cause asphyxia. Channing concluded that the best way was to leave the mask uncovered and keep all lights well away from it. The first clinical fire actually recorded, as far as I know at present, took place in Boston, in July, 1850.[17] The actual cautery was in use near the mouth. The result was not stated.

But it was also found that explosions could occur even when open flames were banned from the operating theatre. They were, of course, traced to static or frictional electricity, which caused sparks of sufficient intensity to ignite inflammable mixtures of gases or vapours. They were fairly common in America, with its dry, continental climate; much commoner than in the damp climate of England.

Ether received a lot of blame as a cause of 'ether bronchitis', especially towards the end of the nineteenth century. This was probably connected with the rise of abdominal surgery from 1880 onwards.

Many people who had fled to ether as a refuge from the uncontrollable and unpredictable treachery of chloroform returned to their first love because of the frequency of 'ether chests'. It began to be realised, however, about the turn of the century, that chest complications depended on other factors as well as—or perhaps instead of—ether. They were far more common in abdominal than in other operations, with the exception of mouth, tongue and jaw cases, which at that time did not have the protection of the respiratory tract from blood and other foreign bodies which is the usual routine today.

It was found, too, especially on the Continent, where the use of local and spinal anæsthetics was far more common than in the English-speaking countries, that the incidence of chest complications remained surprisingly high, again especially in abdominal cases, even though consciousness had never been lost and no irritating substance—in fact no substance of any kind—had been inhaled.

Dr. Gottstein of Breslau[18] reported 233 major operations under Schleich's local infiltration anæsthesia, and commented:

"Affections of the lungs developed as frequently after local as after general anæsthesia produced by chloroform and ether . . . this frequency of pulmonary affections is due, not to the anæsthetic compound, but to the pain which hinders the patient from expectorating."

Again,[19]

"Mikulicz found to his surprise that the occurrence of lung troubles after laparotomy was not in the least affected by employing local instead of general anæsthesia."

Some small scale figures bearing on this point can be given from my own cases anæsthetised in a prisoner-of-war camp in Germany during the Second World War. They are not large enough for statistical analysis, but they are highly suggestive, and they have the advantage that they form an unusually homogeneous group. They were all male adults between twenty and forty years of age, and practically all of them were in very good physical condition, thanks to food parcels sent regularly by the British, Canadian and American Red Cross Societies.

At the stage of the war covered by these figures there was practically no acute war surgery with its attendant mortality. We did have it, earlier and to a lesser extent at the very end of the war—one of the very last anæsthetics I gave was to a badly wounded Waffen S.S. Sturmmann when the American Third Army tanks arrived at the gates of our camp. But for most of the war the operations were largely those of civilian life—hernias, appendixes and so on.

Operating conditions were quite good, though the choice of anæsthetics was somewhat limited. Evipan, open ether, spinals and locals were almost the only available methods. Oxygen we had, but no other gases, except cylinders of butane gas supplied by the Germans for heating the sterilisers. These also came in useful for occasional illicit distillation of a horrible looking liquor produced from fermented packets of Red Cross raisins. (Do not imagine that prison camps were a scene of constant alcoholic excess and debauchery, because you had to save up your weekly packets of raisins for a long time before you had enough to make it worth while to brew up. It only happened on special occasions like Christmas.)

The resultant alcohol was not matured in bond for several years, but drunk as soon as possible in order to escape searches by the German security officers. For temporary stowage I adopted the plan of non-concealment, as advised by Edgar Allen Poe. I kept the alcohol in ether bottles ranged openly in full view on the anæsthetic table. The more enthusiastically ferret-like the searcher the more certain he was to miss something under his very nose. After all, put yourself in his place. Walk into the stark bleakness of an empty operating theatre, rather more sparsely furnished than usual owing to war shortages—and one glance is enough to show you that there isn't any possibility of contraband being concealed there. It is all so blatantly genuine and innocent that the searcher's first instinct is to say, "This is too good to be true. Let us give the doctors' and orderlies' quarters a real good going over. It isn't worth while wasting time here."

In abdominal cases, which includes abdominal wall cases such as hernias, 49 per cent. out of 189 had a cough afterwards. In other types of case only 10·4 per cent. out of 468 had a cough, which clearly shows the difference between the two groups. Nearly all the patients were heavy smokers.

Thirty-nine hernias were repaired under spinal nupercaine; 8 of

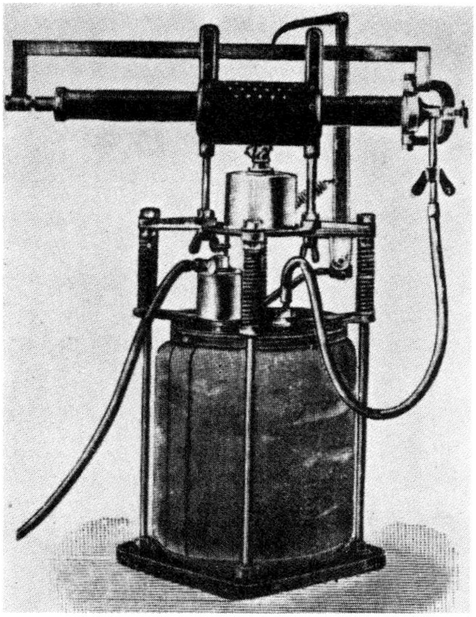

PLATE XXII

Arnold & Sons' Catalogue. 1904, and Lancet, 1902, Oct. 11. 997. L. Kamm & Co.

Medical Oxygen Generator. Produces oxygen when required. Safe and automatic. Weight 25 lb. 12 in. by 15 in. by 23 in. Can be used with spirit lamp or bunsen burner. Retort is of steel. Gas is cheaper than in cylinders. No cylinder carriage to pay. No delay. No danger of explosion as the gas is stored at normal pressure. Cakes of chlorate of potash are heated in a steel retort; the oxygen passes through soda lime into the container, which rises. As the gas is used and the container descends the retort is pulled forward, exposing more cakes to the flame. Another retort can be placed in position without interrupting the supply, when the first is exhausted. Instructions: 1, Open the retort and fill it with oxygen cakes; 2, Replace the retort lid by giving it one or two turns, then put in the screw and suspend the retort over the generator by the hook and pin; 3, Examine the valve. Replace it and screw firmly so that there is no leak; 4, Connect the rubber pipe from container to the retort. Pull retort to the end, so that the first cake is over the flame; 5, Take the purifier off, place piece of wadding in the bottom; half fill it with soda-lime powder; then more wadding, to prevent dust passing. Screw on tightly; 6, Light the lamp; 7, After use take cakes out of retort and clean it with mop and black lead; 8, Oil must not be allowed in the retort or on the rubber container. To make oxygen cakes. Take 4 lb of powdered chlorate of potash and 1 lb black oxide of manganese. Mix, then damp enough to make it hold together. Press in the mould provided. Lay the cartridges to dry in a warm place. One pound of these cakes will fill the retort and produce four cubic feet of gas. The apparatus can be used for making nitrous oxide gas by using the special retort, which is £1 extra.

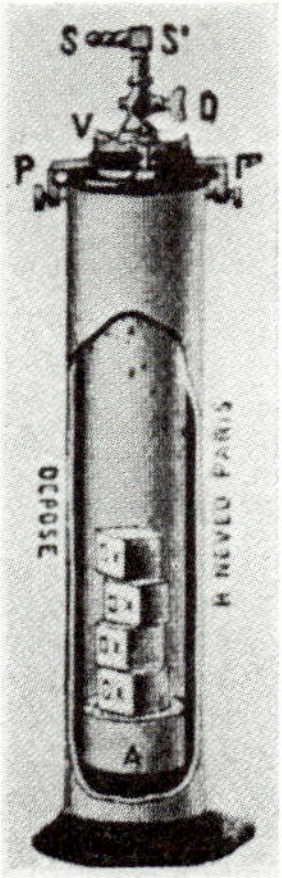

PLATE XXIII

Med. Annu., 1910. 754. Automatic oxygen generator. Adopted by the French Army and Navy. Supersedes cylinders, requires no supervision and no skill. A double cylinder of enamelled iron. The bottom of the inner one is perforated. Sodox cubes (peroxide of sodium) are put in the inner chamber. The outer one is filled with water. When the water and the cubes come in contact pure oxygen is given off, 99·9% pure. Produces 100 litres at one charge. Invented by M. Georges P. Jaubert. Production of gas stops automatically when not in use. Cubes keep well if dry. Always ready for use. No danger of explosion.

Oxygen generators are of two kinds—those in which heating potassium chlorate produces the gas, and those in which water acts on sodium peroxide.

The latter may be made very much lighter than the former—2 lb. as compared to 20 lb., and they are free from fire risk.

An example of each is shown. There are others, such as: *Med. Annu., 1907. 832.* Wollenberg-Draeger generator, and *The Chemistry of Anæsthesia.* John Adriani. 1946. The oxone generator (not dated). Both of these appear to depend on the peroxide process. Also *Brit. med. J., 1909, Nov. 27. 1522.* Leonard Hill, whose apparatus weighs only 2 lb.

"About the beginning of the new century several oxygen generators were introduced, but they did not achieve lasting popularity, which is surprising in view of the weight and bulk of oxygen cylinders."

them had slight coughs and there were 2 cases of pneumonia. Another series of 55 hernias was done under local novocaine block. Of these 17 had coughs and 3 had definite bronchitis.

A small series of 82 appendicectomies was done under three different methods—ether, spinal, and local. There was one pneumonia in 72 ether cases and 2 out of 7 spinals. These series do at least show that pulmonary after-effects are by no means confined to ether anæsthesia, or even to inhalation anæsthesia.

Small as the figures are they interested me and aroused a desire to investigate further. Although the war was now obviously approaching its end I managed to persuade the Germans to supply me with a spirometer. The natural tendency of all men is to go on with the job they are doing until the last possible moment, even when their world is collapsing in ruins about their ears. It was what we had done ourselves when we knew that our hospital was about to be captured by the enemy. In a complex civilisation this is all one can do. It is not possible to drop everything and hide in the jungle, not in Europe anyway. And so it happened, improbable as it may seem, that some surgical instrument maker sent it, the German dispenser received it and passed it on to me, although by that time the Russian guns could be clearly heard from our hospital on quiet nights.

This meant that it was only used in a few cases. I wish I had got it two years before. After all, being a prisoner-of-war has many disadvantages. (This is a masterpiece of understatement.) But it has one advantage and one only, for an anæsthetist. He has plenty of time. Time is the one thing which the prisoner has in abundance. Work was not usually heavy, averaging only about three hours a day, and there were no other distractions. You couldn't go out in your spare time—you had to stop inside the barbed wire. Elderly but nasty-looking machine guns were there to see that you did so. Consequently there was opportunity for investigation, if you could get or make the equipment you needed.

I only had the chance of testing about 20 cases with my spirometer. The end of the war was so near that the Wehrmacht never even got paid for the instrument! Somewhere in the ruins of Hitler's Thousand Year Reich there must be a bill made out in my name for 150 marks or so, but I never got it. Nor did the spirometer survive the war. I took it with me when the Germans evacuated us from the camp in Upper Silesia to the West as the Russian guns drew closer, did a little work with it in the last few weeks and eventually sent it home packed in an old suitcase. But it was squashed beyond repair when it arrived home six months later. After all, spirometers are both bulky and delicate.

Such results as I got were highly suggestive. A series of 9 abdominal and abdominal wall cases showed a post-operative fall averaging 34·7 per cent. of their vital capacity compared with their pre-operative readings. Non-abdominal cases, on the other hand, with the exception of one empyema, did not show any alteration at all. It certainly seemed that interference with the abdominal wall muscles with the consequent splinting effect was the main factor in the production of pulmonary complications.

Ether was still blamed by some surgeons as late as the late 1930s. No doubt it still is blamed in some quarters. Superstitions take a long time to die—almost as long as new ideas take to be born.

Oxygen was first used in anæsthesia about three months after its beginning in England. Mr. James Robinson, the progressive dentist who had collaborated with Dr. Boott in removing Miss Lonsdale's tooth on December 19th, 1846, wrote:[20]

"For the last week I have been using, as a means of resuscitating patients, after inhaling the vapour of ether, pure oxygen gas, with the most perfect success. Today I operated in nine cases on the teeth; to each patient I gave a full dose of the ether vapour, and subsequently a few inhalations of oxygen. In not one case did the patient complain of debility, and all recovered perfectly in less than a minute and a half, timed by the medical men present."

Mr. William Hooper fitted an oxygen attachment to the Robinson inhaler about this date.[21] But it was only rarely employed at this time. Not for very many years did oxygen attachments come into common use. For one thing oxygen was not easy to obtain. It had to be made on the spot, like nitrous oxide. Cylinders of compressed gas did not come into use until 1868, when the firm of Barth put them on the market.[22] In America they were not available until 1871.[23]. About the beginning of the new century several oxygen generators were introduced, but they did not achieve lasting popularity, which is surprising in view of the weight and bulk of oxygen cylinders, even when they became easily obtainable.

Its main employment was in the wards, in cases of severe pulmonary disease, and for years it was given in a very inefficient manner. The old glass funnel waved somewhere near the face was more of a superstitious rite than a practical help in increasing the alveolar oxygen concentration. The fact that the funnel was attached to an oxygen supply at the other end hardly mattered.

But gradually more and more efficient methods came into use and two very surprising things were discovered. It was found that oxygen, which could be taken with impunity at concentrations up to 100 per cent. by ordinary patients, could have disastrous results under two well defined conditions. The gentle, harmless, beneficent and necessary gas, which was an absolute essential to life, had hidden possibilities for evil which had never been noticed before during its use in millions of cases for many decades.

Ninety-five years after Mr. Hooper's oxygen attachment was designed and fitted—in 1942, to be exact—a new condition known as retro-lental fibroplasia was first described by T. L. Terry.[24] It was found that premature infants, especially those who weighed less than 1·5 kg. (3·3 lb.) at birth, were apt to go blind when they were treated in well-equipped, up-to-date hospitals. (It may of course be argued that those who were not treated under these conditions did not live long enough to do the same.) The condition was traced to too-efficient oxygen therapy. It occurred in those who were incubated in high concentrations of oxygen for too long and with sudden discontinuance. The incidence was proportional to the length of the oxygen administration, up to the twelfth day. First of all, dilatation and tortuosity of the retinal vessels occurred, especially affecting the arteries. Then proliferation of the retinal vessels took place, associated with retinal oedema, hæmorrhages and detachment. Then a grey membrane formed at the periphery of the retro-lental space and finally a complete retro-lental membrane formed.

Retrogression could occur after the early stages only. It was found at Bellevue Hospital, New York, that of 36 premature babies who had high (69 per cent.) concentrations of oxygen for at least two weeks, 6 became totally blind. Then, of 28 which received a smaller percentage (38 per cent.) none were affected. A few cases also occurred in the absence of oxygen treatment. An explanation of this may be that the oxygen saturation of arterial blood *in utero* is only 50 per cent., with a rise to 90 per cent. a few hours after birth. This relative increase in oxygen tension might cause abnormal capillary proliferation.

Of 1,999 babies of 4 lb. or under at birth, 1,095 survived for two months, the time required for the condition to develop. Of these, 84 cases (7·7 per cent.) showed the effects; 39 of them regressed, but in 45 there was permanent damage. The condition was not related to the age of the mother, to syphilis, to rubella or to other pregnancy diseases.

An increasing number of cases began to appear in Britain after the Second World War. They followed the introduction of 'efficient' incubators for premature baby units and the use of high concentrations for long periods. The conclusion is that oxygen may be given up to 30 or 40 per cent. for not longer than five days. The condition can be produced experimentally in young kittens by exposure to oxygen, and the effects are proportional to the height of the oxygen tension and the length of exposure.

The condition also varies with the degree of immaturity of the child. Babies weighing 3 lb. 4 oz. to 4 lb. 6 oz. showed an incidence of 0·2 per cent. only, whereas those weighing under 2 lb. 4 oz. were affected in 15·3 per cent. of cases. Children who remained at home appeared to be immune, if they survived.

The second unexpected effect of breathing oxygen only occurs if the oxygen is at a pressure of more than two atmospheres. This is the so-called 'oxygen poisoning' of deep divers and submariners. Sir Robert Davis of the firm of Siebe, Gorman and Co., the manufacturers of diving dresses and breathing apparatus, says in one of his books:[25]

"Oxygen poisoning is another risk to be most carefully guarded against. The breathing of *pure* oxygen above two atmospheres pressure (=33 feet of water), may give rise to nervous symptoms leading to convulsions and blackouts. Its effects are variable, not only in the same individual, but also in different subjects. Warning symptoms are usually stiffening and twitching of the face muscles, but some subjects have no warning and suddenly lapse into unconsciousness. Pure oxygen must, therefore, be avoided for depths beyond, say, 30 feet; for deeper work the oxygen must be diluted in proportion varying with the depths."

This condition can also affect the use of compressed air itself.[26]

"Compressed air cannot be used much in excess of 300 feet because of the danger of poisoning from the oxygen content. . . . At 300 feet, the absolute pressure of the air has increased to ten atmospheres, and, as oxygen forms one fifth of atmospheric air, it will be seen that the partial pressure of the oxygen at this depth is approaching the danger limit of two atmospheres, and that any appreciable increase in depth will subject the diver to the dangers of oxygen poisoning if he continues to breathe compressed air. . . . It is therefore essential that we should use artificial gas mixtures with a reduced oxygen content for deep diving below 50 fathoms."

Paul Bert first showed that oxygen at increased pressures was poisonous to animals. The first human case was in 1912, sixty-five years after the first tentative use of oxygen in anæsthesia. It became an established rule that an exposure of up to three hours at three atmospheres (or 66 feet depth of sea water) was safe. But in training human torpedo oxygen divers in 1942 it was proved that this was not so. The Royal Navy, in conjunction with Siebe, Gorman and Co., carried out experiments which proved that it could be unsafe to dive deeper than 33 feet in sea water. The susceptibility varies even in the same person at different times. The symptoms are pallor, twitching, nausea, dizziness, apprehension, indifference, choking sensations, lights before the eyes, sounds of knocking in the ears and convulsions, which may occur without warning.

This condition, interesting as it is, is outside the scope of anæsthesia. Pressures in anæsthesia are measured in inches of water, not in feet or fathoms, and it is difficult to visualise oxygen poisoning becoming a practical problem in the operating theatre.

Earlier in this chapter I said that ether held the record so far as anæsthetic agents are concerned, with just over three hundred years from its discovery to its first use as an anæsthetic. This is true, but one ancillary drug, and a very important one, though not strictly an anæsthetic agent, had an even longer period in outer darkness.

Curare has been known ever since Hakluyt published his account of Sir Walter Raleigh's voyages in 1595. Charles Waterton, that eccentric but rather charming naturalist, went to South America with the avowed object of obtaining some wourari, as it was then called. This he did, and his adventures in getting it and his experiences with it are worth more than the mere small print footnote which is his fate in those books which mentions him at all. He deserves a special chapter all to himself.[27]

Although curare was used in a few cases of tetanus during the ninteenth century and possibly in a few cases of anæsthesia in the 1920s, H. R. Griffith of Montreal was the first to use it seriously and start it on its career of popularity in 1942, no less than three hundred and forty seven years after Hakluyt's book was published!

But we must not blame the medical profession too much for being slow on the uptake, and for allowing very long latent periods to elapse before new discoveries were put to good use. For a far more astute—and unscrupulous—body of men were also guilty of the same slowness. Cocaine was introduced into medicine by Koller in 1884, but it was not until 1901[28] that the wide boys of racing began to dope racehorses with it. Why the long interval of seventeen years?

References

[1] A. Goodman Levy (1911). *J. Physiol.* Vol. 42. 111.
[2] A. Goodman Levy (1912). *Lancet,* Aug. 24. 524.
[3] A. Goodman Levy (1922). *Chloroform Anaesthesia.* London: Bale & Danielsson.
[4] J. A. Bodine (1903). *Brit. med. J.,* Feb. 21. 446.
[5] *Lancet* (1870), May 21. 737.
[6] Leonard G. Guthrie (1894). *Lancet,* Jan. 27. 193.
[7] George S. Brent (1860). *Lancet,* Sept. 8. 236.
[8] A. Paltauf (1889). *Wien. klin. Wschr.* Vol. 2. 877.
[9] H. H. L. Patch (1922). *Lancet,* Oct. 14. 813.
[10] Kirkby Thomas (1927-28). *Proc. R. Soc. Med.* Vol. XXI. 10. 1705.
[11] W. Stanley Sykes (1930). *Brit. med. J.,* June 21.
[12] G. A. Ibbetson (1868). *Brit. med. J.,* May 30. 548.
[13] A. Coleman (1868). *Brit. med. J.,* Aug. 1. 114.
[14] R. Rendle (1869). *Brit. med. J.,* Oct. 16. 412.
[15] J. H. Humphrey and Margaret McClelland (1944). *Brit. med. J.,* Mar. 4. 315.
S. Carden (1944). *Brit. med. J.,* Mar. 4. 319.
[16] W. Channing (1847). *Boston med. surg. J.* Vol. 36. 366.
[17] *Boston med. surg. J.* (1850), July 31. 538.
[18] *Lancet* (1898), May 7. 1295.
[19] *Lancet* (1904), July 30. 304.
[20] *Lancet* (1847), Apr. 3. 371.
[21] *Pharm. J.* (1847). VI. April. 508.
[22] *Brit. med. J.* (1868), June 27. 635.
[23] Thomas E. Keys (1945). *The History of Surgical Anesthesia.* New York: Schuman.
[24] *Amer. J. Ophthal.* (1942), Feb. 25. 203.
[25] Sir Robert Davis (1955). *Deep Diving and Submarine Operations,* 6th ed. p. 2.
[26] Sir Robert Davis (1955). *Deep Diving and Submarine Operations,* 6th ed. p. 152.
[27] Sykes, W. S. (1960). *Essays on the First Hundred Years of Anæsthesia.* Vol. I, p. 86. Edinburgh: Livingstone.
[28] *Lancet* (1901), July 27. 218.

CHAPTER 7

THE CHEERFUL CENTENARIAN, OR THE FOUNDER OF LARYNGOSCOPY

"The days of our years are threescore years and ten."—PSALM 90. 10.

LORD MOYNIHAN, whose fluency as an orator was equalled only by his lucid prose, wrote an essay on "Truants from Medicine,"[1] in which he described no less than fifty-eight doctors who, for various reasons, became more famous for their work in other fields than in the profession for which they were trained. The article itself is not a good specimen of Moynihan's beautiful literary style, for it is inevitably to some extent a compilation or catalogue, like some of these essays.

He lists revolutionaries like Dr. Guillotine and Jean Paul Marat; statesmen like Clemenceau and Sun-Yat-Sen; administrators of the calibre of Leonard Wood and adventurers like Leander Starr Jameson; writers such as François Rabelais, Conan Doyle and the two Olivers—Goldsmith and Wendell Holmes; Haden the etcher and Livingstone the missionary and explorer.

It occurred to me that it would be interesting to take this idea of Moynihan's and reverse it; in other words, to make a list of men with no medical training who made, or helped to make, spectacular advances in medicine. For example there is Stephen Hales, the Teddington curate who was the first to investigate the blood pressure in animals; there is Charles Waterton, the country squire and naturalist who did so much to rend the veil of secrecy and magic from the mysterious arrow poison curare; and there is Pasteur, whose researches on fermentation paved the way for Lister's antiseptic revolution in surgery. There is the Countess of Cinchon and cinchona bark. None of these were doctors. Nor was the one person in particular who concerns us at the beginning of this chapter.

Manuel Garcia was a famous teacher of singing who wanted, for his own purposes, to examine the vocal cords in action. He succeeded in doing this, and almost casually and quite unwittingly founded a new department of surgery—the department of laryngology. All laryngologists—and they are many—owe their Rolls Royces and their Packards to Garcia. Anæsthetists also owe a great debt to him every time they pass a laryngoscope—or intubate in any other way for that matter. Before Garcia the larynx was *terra incognita*, disregarded completely during life and only seen in the post-mortem room. This is almost but not quite true. Very occasionally intratracheal tubes were passed, by the tactile method, before his time. This was done, in a vain attempt at resuscitation, in the second fatality from chloroform,[2] which occurred less than a fortnight after Hannah Greener's death, and six years before Garcia's first experiments.

A druggist's apprentice, aged seventeen, had contracted the habit of inhaling it. On this occasion when alone in the shop, except for a boy of twelve, he inhaled a large dose and fell forward with his face in the towel on the counter. The boy was frightened to disturb him, as he always became violent after inhaling. Dr. Jamieson intubated the trachea orally and did artificial respiration, but with no effect. But cases like this were very exceptional and quite isolated.

Manuel Garcia[3] was born in Madrid on March 17th, 1805, and died on July 1st, 1906, in his 102nd year. Two of his sisters were famous singers. In 1829 he devoted himself entirely to teaching, and in 1835 he was appointed Professor of Singing at the Paris Conservatoire. He taught Jenny Lind and Charles Santley among many other well known names, and established a great reputation for himself. In 1847 he published *Traité complet de l'Art du Chant*. In September, 1854, he bought a dental mirror from Charrière, the Paris surgical instrument maker, for six francs, which was then worth five shillings or one dollar twenty cents. Was there ever such a large, world-wide business established with such a small capital? He practised with the aid of another mirror until he could see his own vocal cords and find out exactly what they did during the process of vocalisation. On March 22nd, 1855, he read a paper before the Royal Society, "Observations on the Human Voice."

Türck of Vienna was the first to follow up this lead and examine the larynx from the medical point of view, but it was really publicised by Czermak of Budapest. From there the new branch of surgery spread rapidly to every country.

On March 17th, 1905, one hundred years to the day after Garcia was born, a centenary banquet was given, attended by laryngologists from all over the world. Now centenary celebrations are not uncommon: but this one was. It was more than uncommon, it was almost unique, in that the centenarian Garcia himself was present as the guest of honour, and was the life and soul of the party. He was given the C.V.O. by

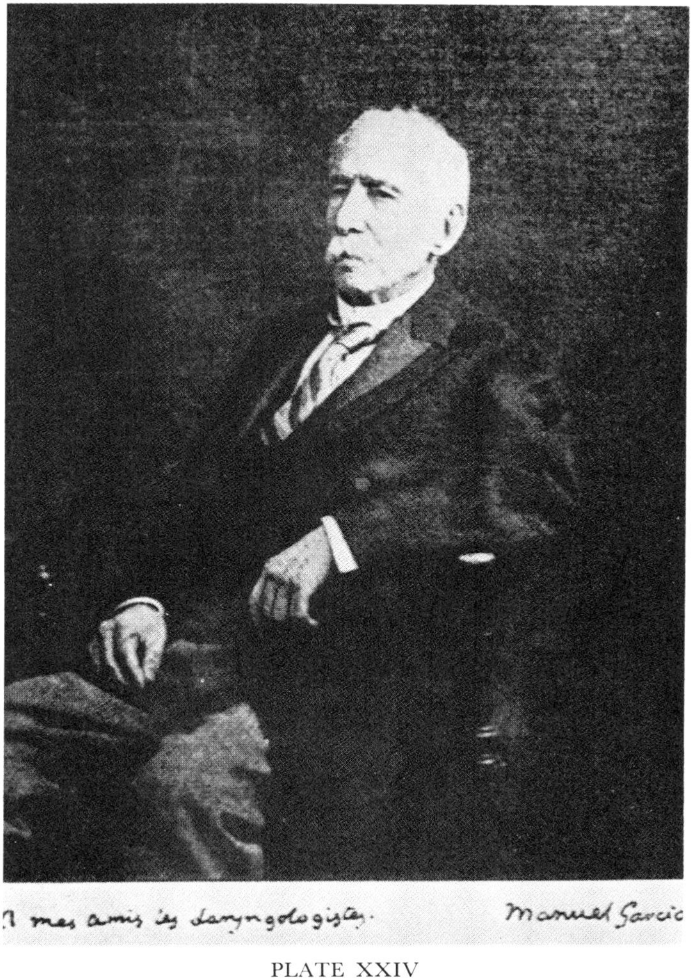

PLATE XXIV

Brit. med. J., 1905, Mar. 25. 681. Manuel Garcia, the founder of laryngoscopy and laryngology. Born in Madrid, March 17, 1805. Died July 1, 1906, in his 102nd year. In September 1854 he examined his own larynx. A famous teacher of singing.

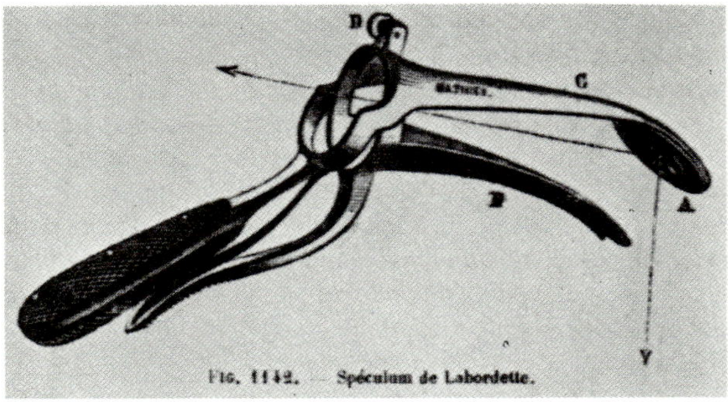

FIG. 1142. — Spéculum de Labordette.

PLATE XXV

Arsenal de la Chirurgie contemporaine. E. Spillman. 1872. vol. 2. p. 527. Spéculum de Labordette.

For an earlier description of this see:

Medical Times and Gazette, 1866, Feb. 24. 213. Dr. Labordette, Lisieux. A bivalve speculum laryngoscope made by S. Maw & Son, in two sizes, 31/- each. A—mirror. It is a mirror, tongue depressor and light conductor in one. This account shows a picture of it in position in a sectioned head.

Edward VII on this occasion, and also received decorations from the Emperor of Germany and the King of Spain.

I have more than 350 pictures illustrating laryngoscopy and laryngeal intubation in relation to anæsthesia, but in view of the high cost of reproduction only a small selection can be given here to illustrate the basic methods and various special points of interest.

There are six different principles involved:

1. Indirect visual laryngoscopy with a forehead mirror and an angled reflecting mirror.

2. Blind oral, tactile intubation. Probably the oldest method.

3. Direct vision laryngoscopy, which involves lifting the tongue and jaw.

4. Blind intubation through the nose with a curved tube.

5. Blind intubation through the mouth, non-tactile, using an introducer.

6. Visual intubation through the mouth, using an introducer, but without lifting.

The first method, indirect laryngoscopy, is virtually that originally used by Garcia, and still used by laryngologists as one of their methods. But it is of little service to anæsthetists, because their interest is not primarily in seeing the larynx but in seeing it in order to pass tubes through it, or even in passing tubes through it without seeing it. The main advantage of the method, that it can be used with a local anæsthetic or even without any anæsthesia, is lost as far as the anæsthetist is concerned, for he practically always has the benefit of general anæsthesia before he uses any laryngeal method at all.

Another disadvantage of this method, for teaching purposes, is that it is difficult for more than one person to see the larynx at a time. Two devices have been described, however, in which this can be done by means of mirrors. Eugen S. Yonge[4] describes, with two very bad photographs, Professor Meyer's (Berlin) apparatus, by which six persons can see the larynx at the same time. Robert M. Lukens, of Philadelphia, pictures an arrangement of angled mirrors above the forehead light[5] which shows an image to an observer on each side of the operator.

Labordette's mirror-speculum is illustrated as an early elaboration of Garcia's method, dating from 1866.[6]

The second principle dispenses with mirrors and vision altogether. Blind, oral, tactile intubation depends on the fact that curved fingers and a curved tube can be passed round the right angled bend at the back of the mouth. It is a method of respectable antiquity, although it was not used very often. The picture is that of Kite's apparatus for the resuscitation of the partially drowned.[7] It was purchased by the the Dumfries and Galloway Royal Infirmary in 1785 and kept at the hospital ready for use.

Laft year, by direction of the Governors, a complete apparatus, or fet of inftruments, ufed for attempting the recovery of perfons *drowned and feemingly dead*, was purchafed. This is to remain conftantly at the Infirmary, ready for immediate ufe; and as there feldom paffes a fummer in which one or more perfons are not loft in the river, perhaps at no great diftance from the Infirmary, it is to be hoped that the means of reftoring fufpended animation, which in many places have been so fuccefsfully practifed, might here likewife prove effectual, if diligently ufed; and if the unfortunate objects, after having been but a *fhort time* under water, be brought *fpeedily* and carefully to the Infirmary.

The wet clothes, if there be any upon it, fhould be eafily and expeditioufly taken off a drowned body, as foon as it is got out of the water. It fhould then be carefully rubbed and dried, and be immediately well covered, either with warm blankets, if thefe can be procured, or with warm clothes and fhirts taken from perfons on the fpot. It is next to be laid eafily in a cart upon ftraw, if there be one at hand, or upon a long broad board, or the like, ftretched out, and upon one fide. In this manner it fhould be carried to the Infirmary with the head and cheft moderately raifed, pretty much in the pofition in which a perfon ufually fleeps, one or more affiftants fupporting the head eafily and fteadily all the way, and taking care that it do not fall too much forwards.

M. Bouchut of Paris,[8] in 1858, constructed a hollow, truncated cone of silver, with a thread fixed to it. He tried this on the dead body and subsequently passed it into the larynges of two live children. The reason is not given, but the probability is that they were diphtheria cases. Dr. Jamieson, ten years earlier still,[2] had done the same, as mentioned above, in an attempt to resuscitate a youth poisoned by chloroform.

Sir William Macewen was born in 1848 and died on March 22nd, 1924, in his seventy-sixth year.[9] He qualified at Glasgow in 1869, just when Lister was preaching his new and startling gospel of cleanliness in surgery. Macewen spent some time after qualification as a resident at the City Fever Hospital, and here he may have got the idea of intubation. He then returned to surgery and became surgeon to the Glasgow Royal Infirmary. He took full advantage of the antiseptic, and later the aseptic, method. Osteotomy, brain surgery, and the complications of otitis

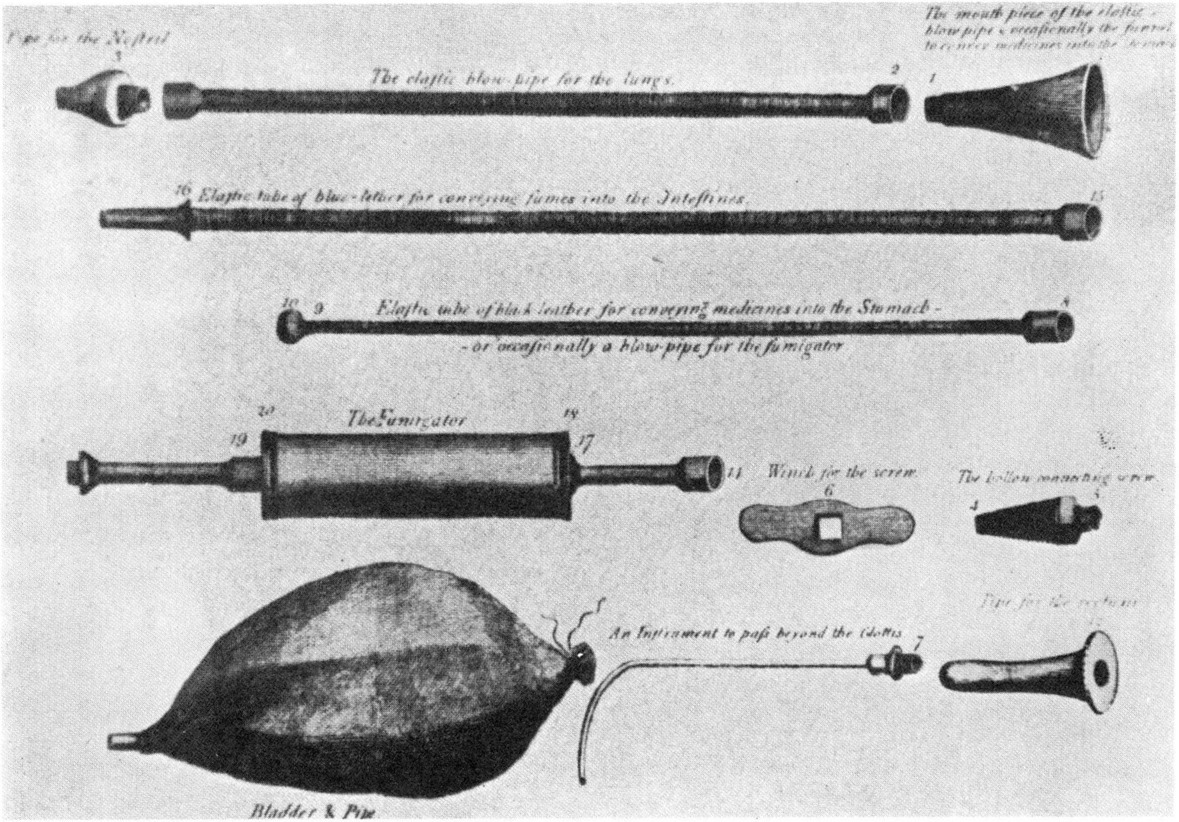

PLATE XXVI

Dumfries and Galloway Royal Infirmary. A pictorial survey. A booklet issued by the hospital in 1948, when it was taken over by the Nationa Health Service. A short history of the hospital as a voluntary institution from 1776 to 1948. Kite's apparatus. Bought by the hospital in 1785. Intended for the resuscitation of the apparently drowned. No. 7 is an intratracheal tube. In addition there are tubes for most of the other orifices of the human body. See text for the full instructions given to the public.

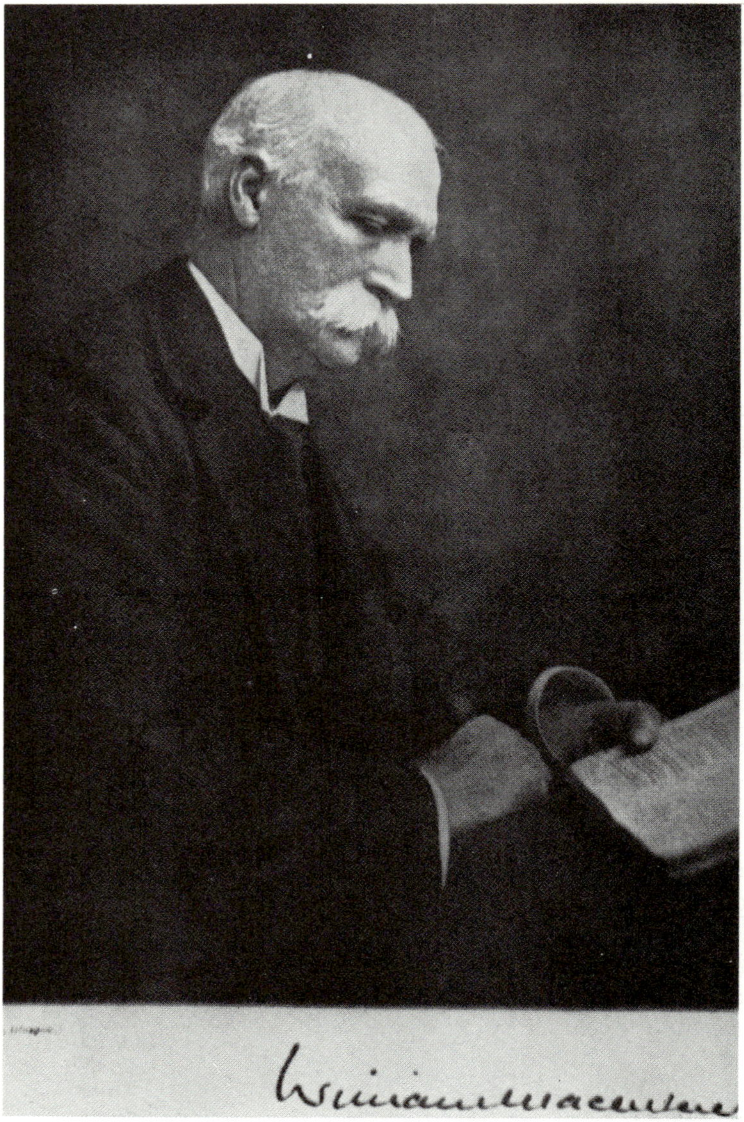

PLATE XXVII

Brit. med. J., 1922, July 29. 175. Sir William Macewen, surgeon to the Glasgow Royal Infirmary. Born 1848. Died March 22, 1924, in his 76th year. First intubated (orally) for anæsthesia July 5th, 1878, in a case of ulcerating epithelioma of the tongue, fauces and pharynx. Successful. He intubated in two more cases for oedema of the larynx. His fourth attempt was again for anæsthetic purposes in a similar case to the first, but the patient died on the table, being ignorant enough not to know that Syme said chloroform was perfectly safe. Macewen described these cases in *Brit. med. J., 1880, July 24. 122,* and *July 31. 163,* in two 5 column articles.

(*By permission of the Brit. med. J.*)

media all engaged his attention, in addition to general surgery. He removed a lung in the early nineties.

He was the first man, I think, to intubate the larynx for anæsthetic purposes, on July 5th, 1878.[10] The patient was a plasterer by trade, fifty-five years old, who had an ulcerating epithelioma of the tongue and right anterior pillar of the fauces, spreading on to the posterior pharyngeal wall.

Macewen, who was thirty years old at the time, had practised oral intubation in the post-mortem room. He described it as much easier than nasal intubation. He rightly thought that this formidable case was very suitable for this method—the only alternative, at that time, being a preliminary laryngotomy or tracheotomy, so as to enable the pharynx to be packed off. The patient was intubated several times before the operation, and it was found that after a little initial coughing he could tolerate the tube quite well. Remember that this was six years before Karl Koller first announced the local anæsthetic properties of cocaine.

So on July 5th he was intubated again, in earnest this time. The cough ceased after a few whiffs of chloroform, long before he was under. Macewen commented that it seemed to have a local sedative action. Dr. Symington, the house surgeon, put him under and a sponge was packed round the tube. It was an extensive operation, starting with sawing through the lower jaw, which was later drilled and wired.

Macewen concluded that chloroform was easily and uninterruptedly given during the whole operation; that there was no interference with the operator; that the breathing was easily heard and felt; that no blood got into the larynx, and finally that the result was excellent.

The next two patients in which Macewen intubated were cases of oedema of the larynx. No anæsthetic was given or intended. The tube was kept in for about thirty-six hours in each case. The patients could swallow with the tube *in situ*.

In the fourth case the tube was scheduled to be used again for anæsthesia. It was another man with epithelioma, who also had bronchitis. Rehearsals were held to see whether he could tolerate the tube. He could—he could even get rid of sputum through it. The tube was put in again and he was taken to the theatre. When the chloroform was started the patient pulled the tube out and asked to be put under without it, saying that it could be put in again when he was under. There was some struggling during induction. Then the case became dramatic.

"Nearly five minutes after the struggle ceased one of the gentlemen who held the radial pulse the whole time, cried out that the pulse had stopped.

The house surgeon said: 'That surely cannot be, as he is breathing all right'. A few seconds later the breathing ceased."

The patient was an ignorant man, who had never heard that chloroform was completely harmless, and he proceeded, most inconsiderately, to die on the table. The post-mortem showed effusion of serum under the arachnoid, and death was attributed to the chronic cerebral affection, the anæsthetic perhaps acting as an exciting cause.

Being intubated without anæsthesia cannot have been very pleasant, but at least the airway was safeguarded and the patient was unconscious of the operation. Only fourteen years before, it will be remembered, Syme still operated in this type of case without any anæsthetic at all—and that was seventeen years after chloroform had been introduced. In fairness it must be remembered that Syme had been used to operating for many years in the pre-anæsthetic era, whereas the span of Macewen's life was wholly within the age of painless surgery. The latter, therefore, could not possibly have developed the protective coating of hard-hearted ruthlessness which the older surgeons had to acquire in order to do their work at all.

Macewen naturally had a completely different outlook. His reflexes were conditioned to anæsthesia, and the idea of major surgery without it was to him unthinkable. And so he was prepared to take trouble in devising and using new methods in order to get the benefit of safer anæsthesia under conditions which made the then routine methods almost impossible and certainly very dangerous.

Possibly this death on the table was responsible for the fact that Macewen did not appear to make any further attempts to spread the new method. He was honest enough to report it, but the death was not exactly a recommendation for it.

It was probably a death from primary heart failure. After all intubation in full consciousness was not the best preparation for chloroform anæsthesia, from a psychological point of view.

The man to whom credit is due for using intubation extensively and publicising it, though not in connection with anæsthesia, was Joseph O'Dwyer, who was born at Cleveland, Ohio, on October 12th, 1841. He qualified in 1866. He held a resident post at the Charity Hospital on Blackwell's Island, and was then appointed physician to the Foundling Hospital in New York in 1872. Here he was horrified at the appalling mortality from diphtheria. It was a common disease in those days, and there was no effective prevention or treatment. Cases in which the diphtheritic membrane spread to the larynx—and this was a matter of luck, for there was no way of stopping it—were generally choked to death by it. And they were so ill that tracheotomy, though it might relieve the obstruction, hardly reduced the death rate at all. Years went by without a single recovery after tracheotomy, and O'Dwyer began to experiment with laryngeal intubation as being a much less severe operation for these moribund patients. He did much research in the post-mortem room and spent endless time making models and casts in order to find out the best shape and size for his tubes. He first used them on the living in 1882, and eventually had a successful case.

He met with the usual opposition at first. All the stock objections to a new idea were brought out once more—that it could not possibly work owing to the intolerance of the larynx for any foreign body; that it wasn't new, anyway, and so on. But it did work; and if it had been done before in occasional cases, what did it matter? O'Dwyer began to save lives with it.

His tubes were small and short[11] and were carried into position on a curved introducer, which was then detached, leaving the tube in the larynx. O'Dwyer died on January 7th, 1898, at the age of fifty-seven. The critics were correct—he had been anticipated in a few isolated cases, as Morton had been anticipated by Crawford Long, but it was O'Dwyer who established intubation firmly and made it widely known.

One of his worries was that many tubes were made and sold which he thought unsuitable; but there is no doubt that detail improvements in his instruments were made. The early tubes needed an introducer and an extractor. Not until later was one unnecessary instrument dispensed with. Instruments were made which could both introduce and and extract, and other tubes were designed which needed no extractor at all. Feroud's is an example of the former,[12] and Hailes's tube[13] one type of the latter.

Another disadvantage of the original pattern, which was overcome in Fischer's modification,[14] was that when the tube was inserted between the cords the patient could not breathe at all until the introducer was removed—and a delay of a second or two was a real and alarming disadvantage to a person who was already half-suffocated. Fischer's tube could be put in and the patient could breathe at once, even before the introducer was taken away. It was the same relation as the old plug bayonet bore to the modern ring fastening—in the former the musket could not be fired when the bayonet was fitted into the muzzle. Fischer's tubes were also corrugated on the outside, so that they were not so easily dislodged. They were made of vulcanised rubber, so they were cheap and a fresh one could be used for each case.

A rather crazy side-line crops up here. Charles L. Greene of St. Paul, Minnesota,[15] designed a very similar tube, which he suggested as a treatment for uncontrollable vomiting. The theory of it was that vomiting is impossible if the vocal cords cannot be closed. He makes no claim to have used his device in practice.

Thomas Annandale, Professor of Clinical Surgery at Edinburgh, progressed far beyond the ideas of his master, Syme. He designed an intratracheal tube "as an aid to certain operations," in 1889.[16] He had it made by Tiemann of New York. It was of stiff elastic material, not too pliable, and had a sliding prop of hard vulcanite to take the pressure of the teeth. It was, of course, curved like a catheter.

O'Dwyer's method was adapted for anæsthetic purposes with great enthusiasm by Franz Kuhn of Kassel.[17] His tube was introduced blindly in exactly the same way and was carried on a curved introducing stilette in order to get round the right angled corner. The difference was that in this case the tube was not merely needed in order to admit air through a choked larynx. An anæsthetic had to be given through it as well. This meant that the short tube was not adequate. The laryngeal part had to be combined with and extended into a flexible metallic tube long enough to reach well outside the mouth, where it ended in a funnel. On this funnel, covered with gauze, ether or chloroform could be dropped. It was really a combination of O'Dwyer's tube and Trendelenburg's cannula, which in its original form was connected to a tracheotomy tube.

Gauze was then packed into the oro-pharynx round the Kuhn's tube, to hold it in position and to prevent the ingress of blood. The anæsthetist then had free access to the lungs and an unrestricted airway, just as in the modern cuffed tube technique.

Kuhn's tube has, and I speak from personal experience, one great and solid advantage over modern methods. It does not depend on dry batteries, which all disappear under the counter in war-time. I used it in about 40 cases in a Kriegsgefangenenlazarett, or prisoner-of-war hospital. My laryngoscope was useless, owing to the absence of batteries, my Magill tubes perished until they were unsafe to use (and the German ersatz rubber tubing was too stiff to make new ones). But Kuhn's tube, being made of flexible metal, was simple, reliable, durable, immutable, imperishable, insusceptible to damage and absolutely indestructible. There was nothing to go wrong, nothing to damage. As a war-time expedient it was excellent.

Kuhn made considerable efforts to publicise his method. He wrote two long articles totalling over 100 pages[17] with twenty illustrations, describing his technique and his tube. In addition to his simple tube he designed an elaborate machine for 'Überdrucknarkose' or pressure anæsthesia, which was fitted with carbon dioxide absorption cartridges. This was in 1906. His machine was fitted with manometers and a water safety valve.[18] He also proposed to fit his simple tube with inflatable laryngeal or pharyngeal cuffs. The only thing he did not do was to design a special gag for the introduction of his tube. Very sensibly he was satisfied with O'Dwyer's.

The third method, of course, is direct vision laryngoscopy, which entails a lifting movement of the tongue and jaw in order to straighten out the right angle so that the cords can be seen. This method split into two divergent techniques. There was suspension laryngoscopy in which the tongue spatula or speculum, usually combined with a gag, hung from a sort of gallows which was attached to or built into the table, and part of the patient's own weight performed the straightening out process against the counter-pull of the spatula. This method was mainly of interest to some surgeons dealing with the larynx and the air passages beyond it. It was largely used by Killian, one of the pioneers.[19] But it was no use to the anæsthetist, who required something more portable, something which could be picked up, used quickly and laid aside. The gallows was too cumbersome, too permanent and too structural for their modest requirements.

And so the ordinary hand laryngoscope was developed by a host of individuals, amongst whom should be mentioned Chevalier Jackson.[20, 21] His gentleness and dexterity were so great that he usually dispensed with general anæsthesia, even for bronchoscopies. He relied on skilled positioning of the patient's head by a well trained and intelligent assistant, in preference to the rather brutal and unintelligent fixed pull of the suspension gallows. But from the fact that Jackson described, and presumably sometimes used, a sort of bite block and finger protector, it would appear that even the maestro himself occasionally ran into trouble.[22]

Chevalier Jackson was born on November 4th, 1865, and qualified at Philadelphia. He became Professor of Laryngology at Pittsburgh in 1912. In 1916 he was appointed Professor of Bronchoscopy and Oesophagoscopy at the Jefferson Medical College, Philadelphia. His experience in removing foreign bodies from the bronchi of inquisitive children was enormous, because for many years he had little competition in this sort of work. He died on August 16th, 1958, at the age of ninety-two.

The direct vision laryngoscope at first had no light at all attached to it. It was used in conjunction with an electric light reflected down the lumen by a prism (Killian). Distal illumination was then fitted, as in Jackson's early models.[23] For a long time this meant the inconvenience of trailing wires leading to a separate battery box, which nuisance was in production as late as 1932,[24] though in this particular model the inconvenience was lessened by the cord passing through the hollow handle of the instrument. Eventually the battery was housed in the handle, making the whole thing self-contained and much easier to handle.

Laryngoscopes were at first shaped like three sides of a square, with a lifting handle parallel to the spatula, which perhaps made it easier to expose the larynx without leverage on the front teeth. The three sides were then cut to two—merely a spatula and a combined handle and battery container. There were wide varieties in the way the spatula was fastened to the handle, many models having a right angle, others an acute angle,[25] and others again an obtuse angle,[26] which suggests that the size of the angle itself is of little importance, though MacBeth and Bannister claim that their obtuse angle abducts the wrist and discourages leverage on the front teeth.

The first laryngoscope designed with a slightly curved blade was put forward by Janeway in 1913.[27] Miller[28] and Cassels[29, 30] also used a similar design in 1941. Wiggin produced another in 1944.[31] In this one the curve was confined to the tip of the blade only. These were all suggested on the ground that the traditional straight-bladed pattern was designed to allow the passage of the rigid, straight tube of a bronchoscope rather than a curved flexible tube, as generally used in anæsthesia. Moreover they were all used in the traditional way—whether straight or curved—that is, they were passed beyond the epiglottis before they were lifted, and the curves were all quite slight.

Macintosh[32] brought out a scope with a hooked end to the blade to act as an epiglottis retractor. It also had the advantage of using an ordinary cheap flashlight bulb instead of the usual tiny and expensive surgical lamp. The extra bulk of this meant that the lamp could be not distally placed, but the light was conducted distally through a curvlite or lucite light-conducting plastic rod.

Less than two years later, however,[33] Macintosh swung to the other extreme. From an epiglottic retractor he passed on to a new and more original instrument still, which disregarded the epiglottis. Its very short, sharply curved blade was specifically designed to avoid hooking it up. The blade was passed into the glosso-epiglottic recess, and it was found

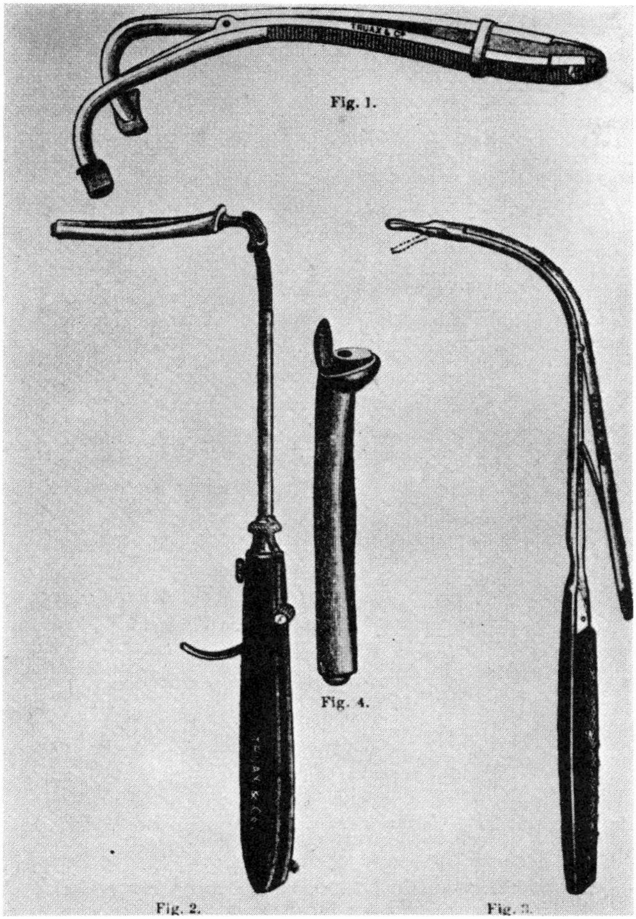

PLATE XXVIII

Brit. med. J., 1888, Sept. 29. 716. F. E. Waxham, Chicago. O'Dwyer's intubation set. These pictures (Plates xxviii and xxix) were chosen out of many because they show all the essentials and because of the charming little picture showing how the tubes are used.

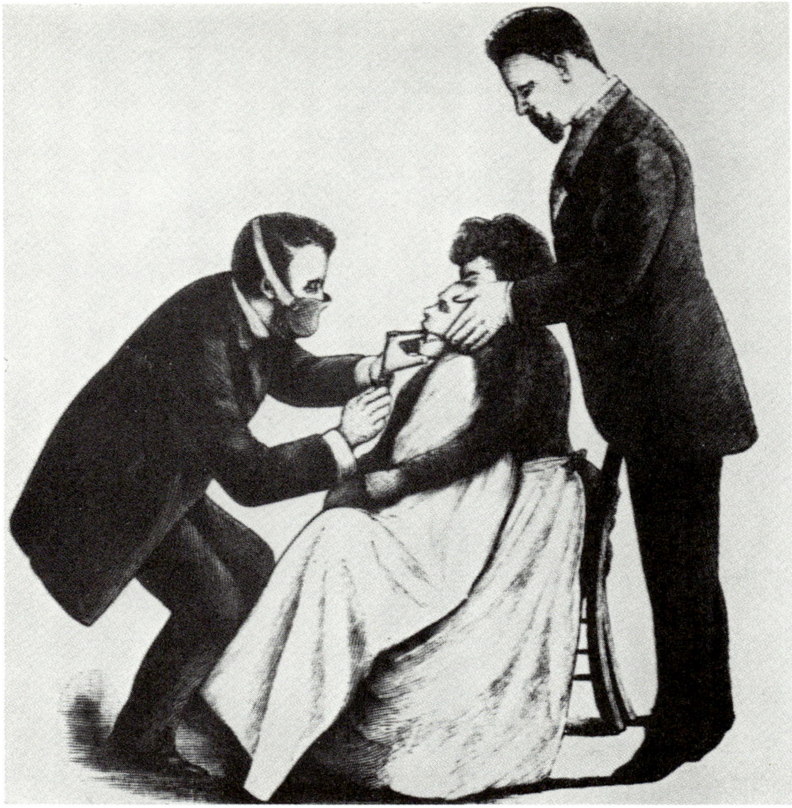

PLATE XXIX

Brit. med. J., 1888, Sept. 29. 716. F. E. Waxham, Chicago. O'Dwyer's intubation set. These pictures (Plates xxviii and xxix) were chosen out of many because they show all the essentials and because of the charming little picture showing how the tubes were used.

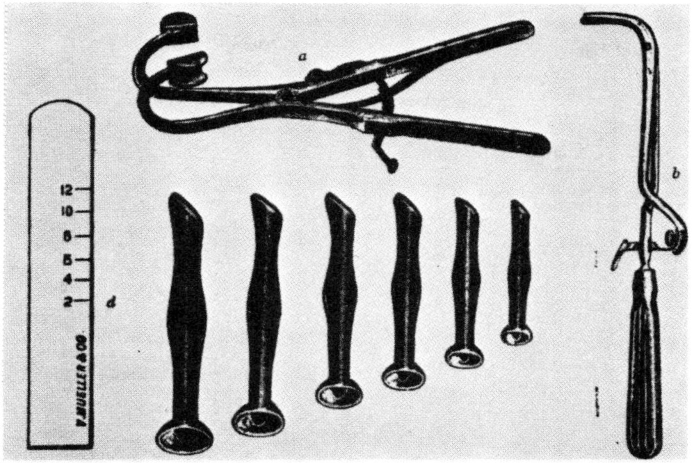

PLATE XXX

Med. Rec. N.Y. 1912, Jan. 6. 17. Abraham Levinson, Chicago. Feroud's intubation set. *a*, gag; *b*, introducer and extractor combined. This is an improvement on the original pattern, which required separate introducers and extractors; *c*, gold-plated metal tubes; *d*, scale of years for measuring the sizes of the tubes. Very useful for the non-expert, one would think.

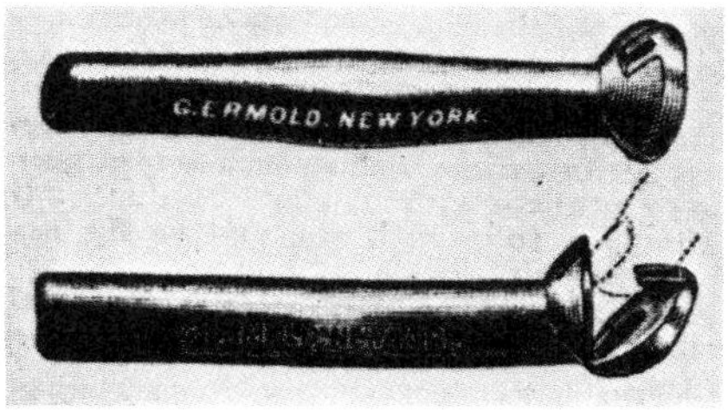

PLATE XXXI

Brit. med. J., 1890, May 24. 1187. William Hailes, Albany, N.Y. Modified and improved O'Dwyer's tube, which can be removed without an extractor.

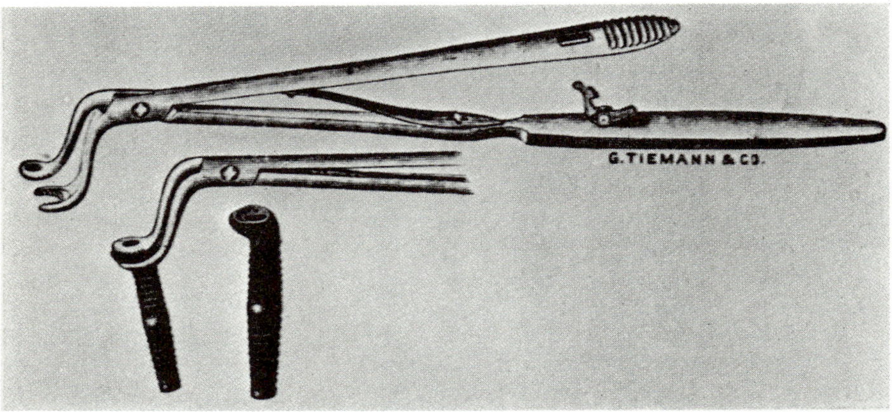

PLATE XXXII

Med. Rec. N.Y., 1897, June 19. 873. Louis Fischer, New York. Modified O'Dwyer's tubes. Made by Tiemann & Co. They are made of vulcanised indiarubber. They are cheap and a fresh one can be used for each patient. The corrugations on the outer surface prevent the tube from being easily dislodged. The introducer does not block the lumen of the tube, as it did in many models.

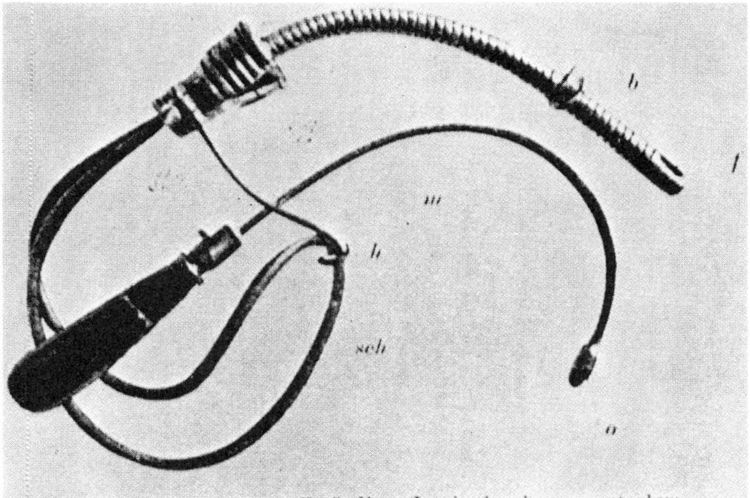

Fig. 2. Mein jetziges vollständiges Intubationsinstrumentarium.

PLATE XXXIII

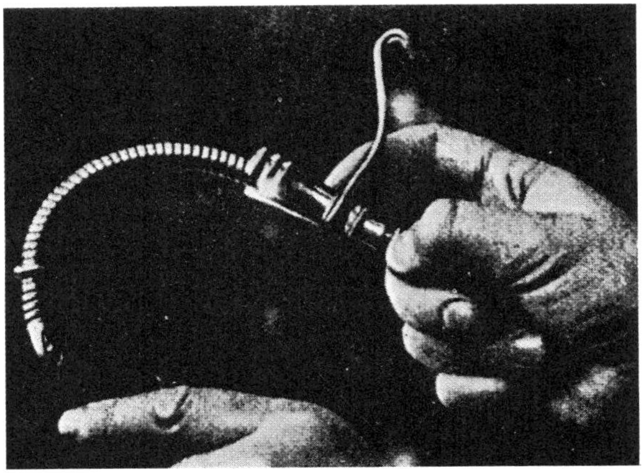

PLATE XXXIV

PLATES XXXIII and XXXIV

Arch. Klin. Chir., 1905. 76. 148-207 and *1905, 78. 467-520.* Franz Kuhn. Kassel. Selected from the 20 illustrations in these two long articles.

" . . . my present complete intubation armamentarium." Sch—schlauch or elastic tube to tie round the neck. This is not necessary when the tube is packed into position with gauze.

" . . . method of introduction." The wire contraption above the right index finger is not fitted to my Kuhn's tube. Mine is also more pointed at the laryngeal end, which makes for easier introduction.

Neither of these pictures shows the extension tube, which fastens on with a bayonet joint and has a funnel at the other end. It is about the same length as the tube itself.

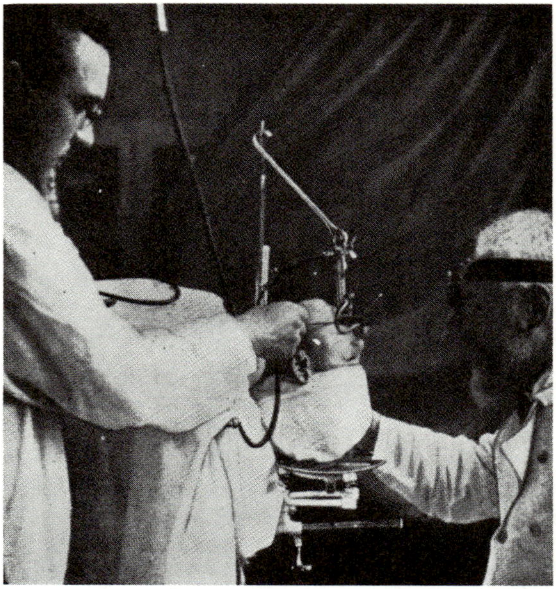

PLATE XXXV

Med. Annu., 1915, plate XXX. Suspension apparatus in position with Junker's apparatus connected up. The man with the beard is Killian himself.

(By permission of the publishers)

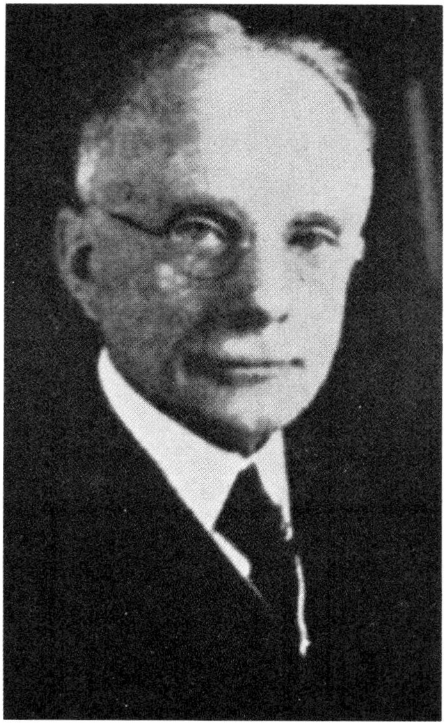

PLATE XXXVI

Brit. med. J., 1958, Aug. 30. 568. Chevalier Jackson. Obituary. The picture shows him at the age of 65 (about 1930). " . . . safe and routine bronchoscopy was entirely due to him." He made his own instruments and streamlined the ponderous apparatus of Killian and Brünings. He had tuberculosis and had long absences from work, which he occupied by writing textbooks on his own subject. In spite of his complaint he lived to be 92.

(*By permission of the Brit. med. J.*)

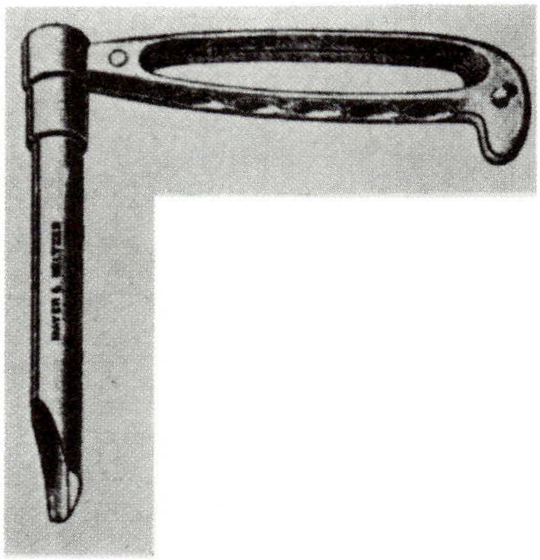

PLATE XXXVII

Med. Annu., 1908. 168. Killian's tube spatula
No light attached.

that lifting in this position gave satisfactory exposure. It was claimed that it could be used under lighter anæsthesia and that there was less risk of damage to the teeth, owing to its completely open top. There was also less risk of damage to the posterior pharyngeal wall, as the blade could be kept in close contact with the tongue during its whole passage. A lateral tongue guard was fitted to prevent the tongue obscuring the view.

The originator explained[34] that the shape of the blade did not matter very much, provided that it did not pass beyond the epiglottis. A straight blade was better for passing a straight tube and vice versa.

Many refinements came into being through different inventors. A hinge was introduced so that the blade could be folded flat against the handle. This made the instrument easier to pack. But a bigger advantage was the automatic switch incorporated in the hinge which put the light on when, and only when, the blade was lifted into its working position.

Other models had interchangeable blades of different sizes, while some were built especially for infants and children. G. F. Gibberd and J. B. Blaikley[35] used a small one for the treatment of asphyxia neonatorum, and Alan Moncrieff[36] described a slightly different model of Gibberd's. The Shadwell scope for infants was illustrated by Noel Gillespie in his excellent book.[37] Robert A. Miller[38] designed a very small instrument, for visualisation of the larynx only. The tube was introduced outside the blade. Phyllis Daplyn[39] used a special model for babies with cleft palates—the blade being very broad so that it did not slip into the cleft.

A very unusual shape was suggested by MacBeth and Bannister.[26] In addition to the obtuse angle formed by the handle, which has already been mentioned, the handle itself was offset to a considerable extent. The appearance was ungainly, however good the apparatus was to handle; it rather resembled a gun built for the right shoulder of a left eyed shooter. No gunmaker, however skilful, can make one of these beautiful, or anything but lopsided.

Lundy[40] gives a picture of Seldon's blade for his own (Lundy's) laryngoscope. This is very thin and can be used when it is not possible to open the mouth fully. A similar instrument with a very thin blade was devised by James A. Bennett[41] for use in cases of Ludwig's angina. He pointed out that the mortality of these cases is very high—50-60 per cent.; that blind intubation usually fails because of oedema of the larynx and its surroundings, and that ordinary laryngoscopes cannot be used because the mouth cannot be opened widely enough. His scope has an acute angled, thin, flat blade which is scarcely more than a tongue depressor.

It seems to me that a special instrument of this kind, though it would only be used very rarely indeed, might be an invaluable life-saver in these difficult and dangerous cases. In the old days they were responsible

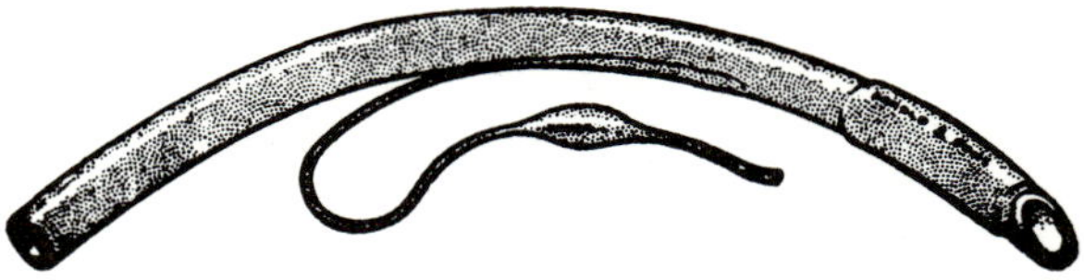

MAGILL'S ENDOTRACHEAL TUBES

For large animals. With inflatable cuff and pilot balloon.

Sizes available:—

	Internal Diameter	Length
1	5/8"	2' 0"
2	·3/4"	2' 6"
3	7/8"	2' 6"
4	1"	2' 10"

FIG. 11

Arnold & Sons, London. Catalogue of Instruments. 1954. Magill's tubes. How very ordinary! Why put in a picture of something which is a common object in every operating theatre?

Quite, but these tubes, though it is not obvious, are a little unusual. A table of sizes accompanied them in the catalogue. Size 4, the largest, was 2 feet 10 inches long and 1 inch internal diameter! You see, Arnold & Son make only veterinary instruments, and these tubes are for large animals.

for most of the deaths which took place under nitrous oxide. It was not realised for many years that they were actual or potential cases of severe respiratory obstruction; that the patient was forced to use his accessory muscles of respiration in order to breathe at all; and that, as soon as these voluntary efforts were suspended by anæsthesia, effective respiration ceased at once. Matters were made even worse, if possible, by the congestion of pure nitrous oxide—for gas was known to be safe, and 'a whiff of gas' long enough to open an abscess couldn't hurt anybody. But it

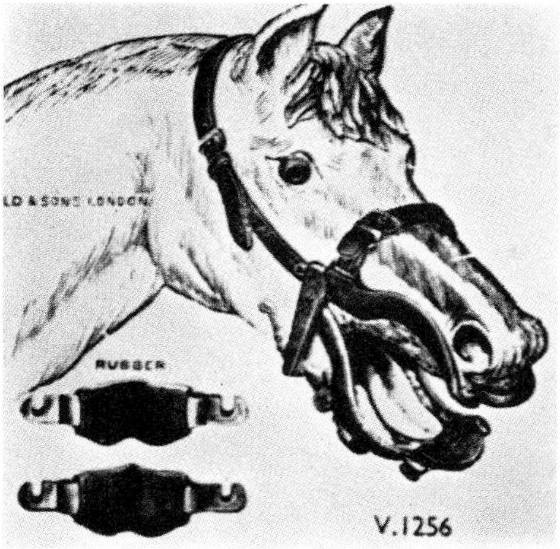

PLATE XXXVIII

A few more mouth gags from a large selection, showing the sort of gag that might be used for insertion of the immense Magill tubes mentioned above, and the sort of patients on which they are used. This is the elimax gag.

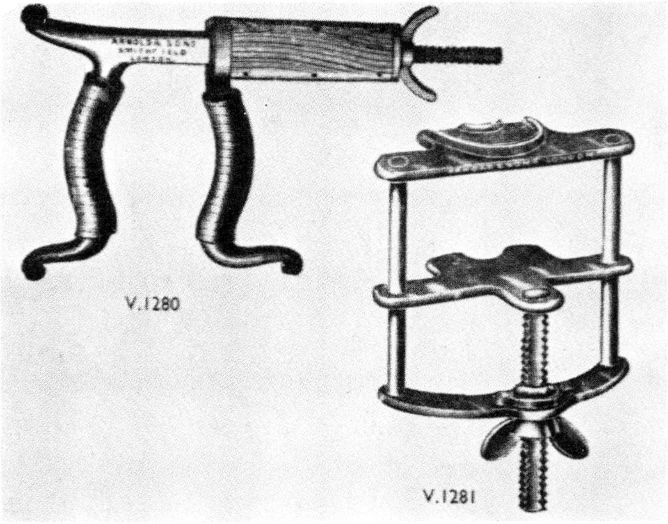

PLATE XXXIX

Two more gags, adjustable this time. V1280 is Varnell's with rubber covered jaws; V1281 is Butler's extra strong. All the above, of course, are from Arnold's Veterinary Catalogue. 1954.

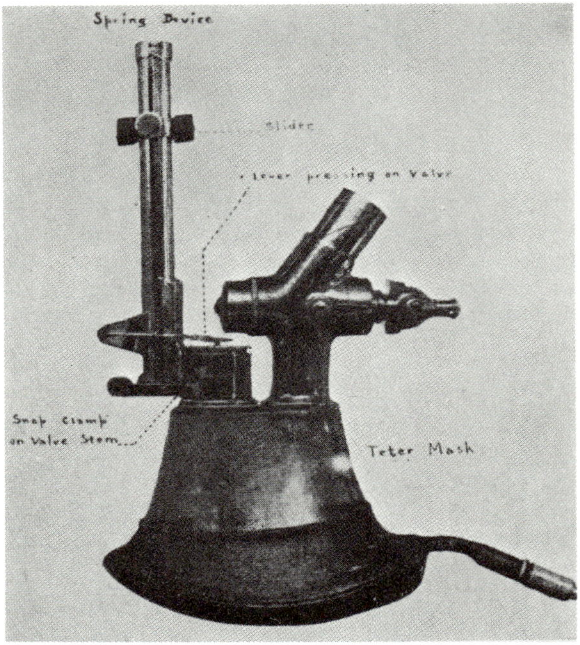

PLATE XL

J. Amer. med. Ass., 1912, Mar. 23. 836. Sterling Bunnell. San Francisco. Positive pressure gas oxygen for thoracic surgery. $4\frac{1}{2}$ column article. An adjustable spring device clamps on to the expiratory valve of Teter's mask. The pressure is adjusted by the slider. The pressure prevents collapse of the lung in operations on the thorax. It is the only special apparatus needed for positive pressure.

Its simplicity will be appreciated on comparing it with Morriston Davies's formidable machine.

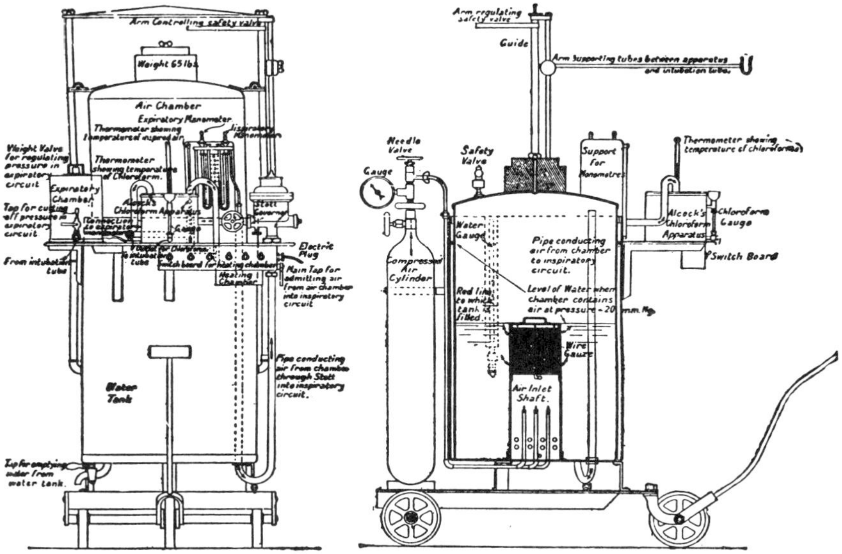

PLATE XLI

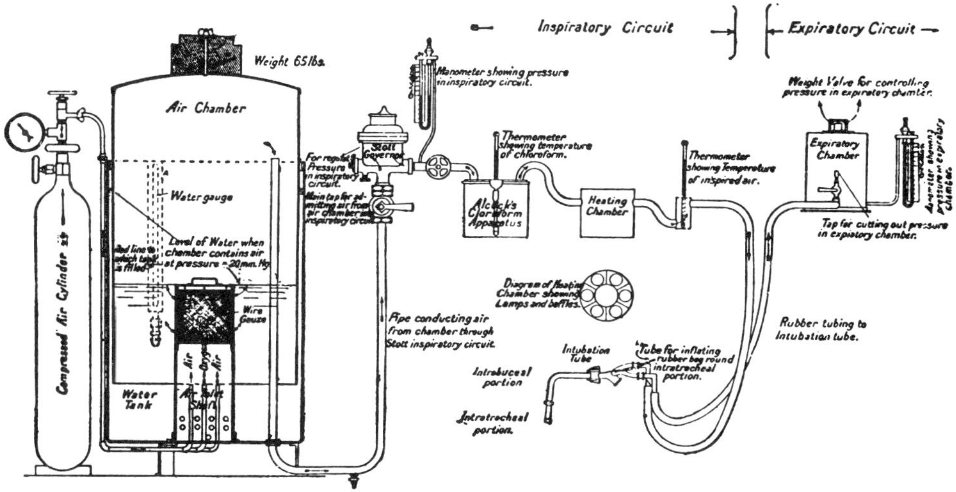

PLATES XLI, XLII

See Legend attached to Plate XLIII

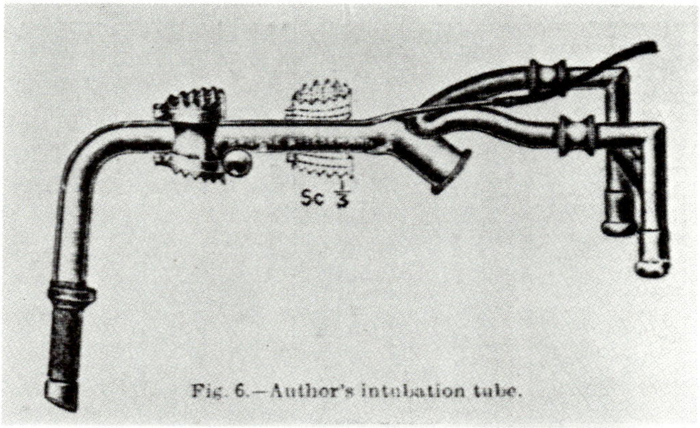

PLATE XLIII

Brit. med. J., 1911, July 8. 61. H. Morriston Davies. Assistant surgeon, University College Hospital. 11 column article on the mechanical control of pneumothorax during operations on the chest. Davies's hyper-atmospheric apparatus. The air pressure remains constant, but can be varied. Simple to use. No motors. Transportable (in what?). Efficient. Can be used in any operating theatre. It was used for Morriston Davies by Felix Rood.

In the picture of the intubation tube note the sliding tooth block, and the inflatable cuff with the small tube leading from it.

Now do you see why I referred to a "monstrous spate of machines of increasing elaboration and complexity"?

(*By permission of the Brit. med. J.*).

could, and it did, in these cases. Bennett further advised that the tube should be left in position for twenty-four hours, to allow the oedema to subside.

In the early 1920s Ivan Magill introduced a fourth method of intubation—the blind passage of a curved rubber tube through the nose. This was quick and convenient, and if it failed, as it occasionally did even in the hands of experts, it could always be helped out by a scope and a pair of curved forceps, which could pick up the recalcitrant tube in the pharynx and guide it into position. And this simple method cut out the use of the laryngoscope with its possibilities of trauma, in a large percentage of cases. Macewen had tried this method in 1878 but abandoned it in favour of oral intubation, which he considered easier. Probably the nasal tubes he tried had not a sufficient or permanent curve.

It would not ordinarily be worth while to show a picture of such a common object as a Magill's tube, which is part of the equipment in every operating theatre.[42] But the picture given is really a little out of the ordinary. In the original there is a table of the four sizes in which these tubes are made. The largest is 2 ft. 10 in. long and one inch internal diameter; the smallest is 2 ft. long and $\frac{5}{8}$ inch diameter! The picture is taken from Arnold and Sons' Catalogue of Veterinary Instruments. With the tubes are shown a few of the many gags which might be used for the insertion of these colossal tubes.

When I was collecting photographs of anæsthetic apparatus on a large scale, in addition to getting them from the pages of the medical journals, if possible with the original author's remarks, I also borrowed catalogues from various surgical instrument makers. One of the firms I wrote to was Arnold and Sons, who used to have a showroom, if I remember rightly, just opposite St. Bartholomew's Hospital. I believe I bought my first stethoscope there. They informed me that they now made veterinary instruments only, but offered to lend me their sole remaining copy of their old complete catalogue of (human) instruments. As it was very heavy it was sent to their York branch, and I collected it there. It was a huge book, nearly seven inches thick. It contained nearly 2,000 pages of heavy calendered shiny paper, with nearly 6,000 illustrations. It was difficult to handle for the camera; the book was so thick that the pages would not lie flat. By internal evidence it was later than 1901, but not much later. A photograph of the firm's grinding department showed bare grindstones with no dust removal hoods. The preface said that the firm was established in 1819, 'Nearly a hundred years ago.' Finally the date was found to be 1904. I also borrowed one of their current catalogues of veterinary instruments and found in it various items of interest concerning animal anæsthesia.

The very earliest intratracheal methods were by means of two way tubes through which the patient breathed in and out. Macewen's tube and Kuhn's tube were both on this simple principle. Then, with the development of the early laryngoscopes, insufflation methods became popular. A gum elastic catheter was passed through the cords by direct vision, and a current of air carrying with it the anæsthetic vapour was blown into the lungs, the return current escaping round the tube. This exhaust current was relied upon to prevent the entrance of blood. The insufflation era began about 1912, when Boyle and Gask[43] designed a simple apparatus for blowing air over ether by means of a foot bellows. Then there burst upon the world a monstrous spate of machines of increasing elaboration and complexity, in which electric motors drove a fan which blew air down the catheter. All these mechanical horrors had to be provided with manometers to measure the working pressure and with blow off safety valves in order to avoid distending the patient beyond repair. Kelly's[44] apparatus in 1912 was followed by Salzer's[45] and Elsberg's[46] in 1913 and many others.

About 1922, ten years or so after the insufflation extravaganza began, Magill's new method of nasal intubation restored some of the old simplicity to endotracheal anæsthesia, although insufflation machines continued to be designed and sold up to about 1930. It was found that tubes large enough for two way traffic could be passed through the nose, and although complex machines continued to be used to supply the various mixtures required, they were no longer essential. The old Kuhn funnel or the 'tin can' method could be used. There was no real need to blow the gases at the patient when a wide tube was used—the patient could perfectly well help himself.

The differential pressure chambers of Sauerbruch (1904), illustrated by Mushin and Rendell-Baker,[27] developed into the still more impressive and enormously expensive specially built pressure operating theatres described by Willy Meyer in 1909 and 1911.[47, 48]

Then there came a sudden blast of shattering simplicity, which was long overdue. In 1912 Sterling Bunnell[49] of San Francisco fixed a small adjustable spring pressure device on to the expiratory valve of a Teter gas-oxygen mask. This was about the size of a penknife, and Bunnell claimed that it would maintain control of the respiration when the chest was open.

Inflatable cuffs on tracheal tubes became very popular as a liquid-

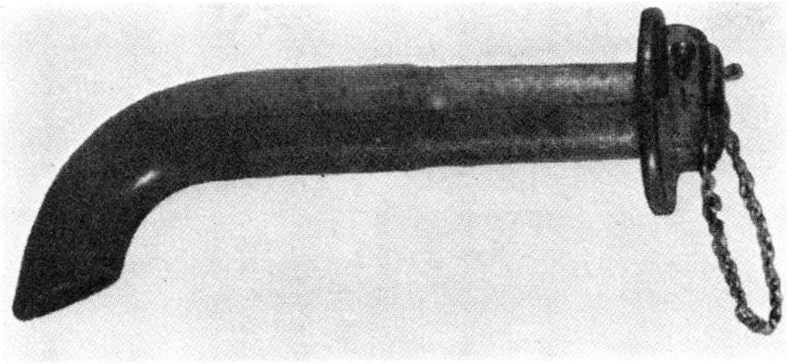

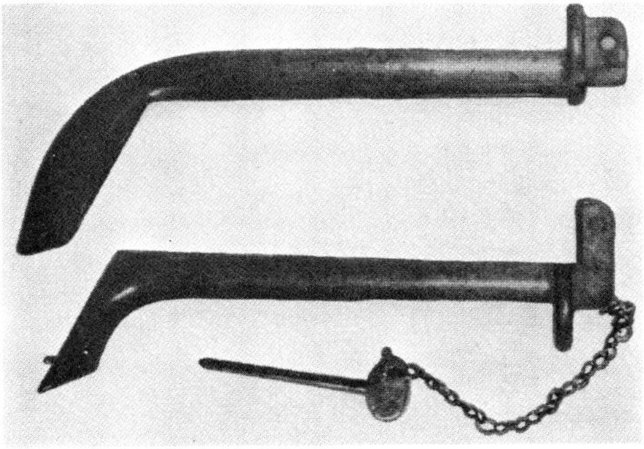

PLATES XLIV and XLV

The divided airway.

tight seal to safeguard the airway. They were merely a revival of the cuff suggested by Kuhn[17] in 1905 and Morriston Davies in 1911.[50] A self-inflating cuff was designed by Mushin and reported by Macintosh.[51] A hole in the side of the tube, covered by the cuff, allowed the gases in the tube to fill the cuff. It was as simple as that.

Most cuffed tubes were too bulky to be passed through the nose, and they had to be inserted through the mouth with the aid of a laryngoscope. But Grimm and Knight[52] produced a tube with a very thin cuff which could be used for nasal intubation.

Cuffs could become deflated, so a pilot bag connected to the cuff but left in full view outside the mouth was added, to give warning of this mishap, if it occurred.

At least one death was caused through the bursting of a cuff, with consequent rupture of the trachea.[53] Is there any device in the whole of anæsthesia which has not killed somebody?

The fifth method is blind intubation through the mouth, but non-tactile this time. An introducer is used to guide the tube in the direction of the larynx. An ordinary Magill tube, or a special central pointed tube is simply passed through a divided metal airway.[54] This, which is rather longer than an ordinary airway and with perhaps a slightly more acute bend, is just as easy to insert. When it is in the anæsthesia can be deepened, if necessary. This ability to split the manœuvre into two parts is of great value when relaxants are not available. The tube is then pushed into the airway, moved about a little until the maximum blast of air is coming through it and then pushed home, preferably during an inspiration. Personally I find this method more frequently successful than nasal intubation—but it does fail occasionally. About once in seventy times, according to my records. It is quicker and simpler than any other method and less traumatic (or it was, in pre-relaxant days).

After the tube is in the trachea, the airway can be split into two halves by removing a pin, and the halves removed separately. The pin is chained to one half for security.

A somewhat similar device was designed by Mark I. Knapp in 1896,[55] the difference being that Knapp's director was made for the passage of a stomach tube. Its curve is consequently less acute. Knapp records, two years later,[56] that he had used it successfully in 4 cases in which the passage of a stomach tube without it had failed.

Mushin and Rendell-Baker give illustrations of two other devices which resemble the divided airway more closely, for they were both intended for directing tubes into the trachea. One, Leroy's introducer

(1827)[57], was old, much older than anæsthesia, and the other, Crafoord's introducer of 1938,[58] fairly modern.

One other possible method remains, which has not to my knowledge been previously used or described. It combines the speed and simplicity in use of the divided airway with the reliability given by vision and a complete absence of lifting or straightening out of awkward angles. I thought of this method as a prisoner, when intubation was sometimes difficult.

I suppose that with relaxants laryngoscopy is invariably easy nowadays, but it was not always so. It could be very awkward at times, especially with a tough and muscular patient, in the days when nothing but deep anæsthesia would relax the jaw. Sometimes it was almost impossible to attain this at the beginning of the anæsthesia, when it was most needed.

A divided airway could be modified by casting two small side tubes as an integral part of it. These would stop short at the angle and the airway would not be any more difficult to introduce. Its breadth from side to side would be a little greater, but this does not matter—its depth would be unchanged, and it is on the depth, and the amount of jaw opening it needs that ease of introduction depends. Down one side tube is a source of light, probably through a curvlite or lucite rod. In the other is a series of lenses and an angled mirror, somewhat like a periscope.

Then, merely by inserting an airway and switching on the light the larynx would be visible 'round the corner', without any lifting at all, and the tube could be passed through the airway and seen to pass between the cords. It somewhat resembles Labordette's principle. The lenses could be arranged to give an upright image.

This device, though attractive and just what was wanted for the somewhat crude working conditions as a prisoner, was too complicated to be made in the camp. When I got home I dropped the idea for two reasons; first, I gave up anæsthesia, and secondly, I thought that the introduction of relaxants had probably made it unnecessary. If I am wrong and such a contrivance would still be of help, it is not patented and anybody is at liberty to make it and use it. I included it here for the sake of completeness, as the principle is somewhat different from all the other methods. There is no reference number, as it has never been published.

Accessories for endotracheal anæsthesia are without end. There is no living anæsthetist who holds the distinction of *not* having designed one or more. They range from clips and fastenings of all kinds to hold the tube in position, to curved tin boxes (and later curved plastic containers) in which to store tubes at their proper curvature; from gadgets for fitting cuffs on to tubes to the old double-channelled catheters of the days of insufflation, to spare the surgeon the blast of ether-laden air from the lungs of the patient; from holes to slots—holes in Ayre's semi-open method[59] and slots in Frank Cole's slotted tube,[60] which allows free breathing by both lungs even if it is inadvertently pushed into the right bronchus by mistake; from spiral wire tubes to transparent plastic;[61, 62] from cleaning brushes to connecting pieces which allow for suction to be used.

Bronchoscopes have developed from the clumsy instruments of Killian to those with an attachment for a cine-camera,[63] and those which can be used anywhere at any time without the elaborate set-up of a bronchoscopy clinic. Two models[64, 65] of an emergency bronchoscope have appeared, with a dry battery in their handles.

References

[1] Lord Moynihan of Leeds (1936). *Lancet,* May 30. 1254.
[2] Dr. Jamieson (1848). *Lancet,* Feb. 19. 218.
[3] Manuel Garcia (1905). *Brit. med. J.,* Mar. 25. 681.
[4] Eugene S. Yonge (1904). *Lancet,* Apr. 30. 1195.
[5] R. M. Lukens (1927). *J. Amer. med. Ass.,* Dec. 17. 2113.
[6] *Med. Times and Gaz.* (1866). Feb. 24. 213, and E. Spillman (1872), Arsenal de la Chirurgic contemporairie. Vol. 2. 527.
[7] Dumfries and Galloway Royal Infirmary. 1776-1948. A Pictorial Survey.
[8] M. Bouchut (1858). *Lancet,* Oct. 2. 364.
[9] Sir William Macewen (1922). *Brit. med. J.,* July 29. 175.
[10] *Brit. med. J.* (1880), July 24. 122.
Brit. med. J. (1880), July 31. 163.
[11] F. E. Waxham (1888). *Brit. med. J.* Sept. 29. 716.
[12] *Med. Rec. N.Y.* (1912), Jan. 6. 17.
[13] *Brit. med. J.* (1890), May 24. 1187.
[14] *Med. Rec. N.Y.* (1897), June 19. 873.
[15] *Med. News* (1895), July 6. 9.
[16] *Brit. med. J.* (1889), Mar. 2. 465.
[17] Franz Kuhn (1905). *Dtsch. Z. Chir.* Vol. 76. 148.
(1905). *Dtsch. Z. Chir.* Vol. 78. 467.
[18] Franz Kuhn (1906). *Dtsch. Z. Chir.* Vol. 81. 63.
[19] Gustav Killian (1920). *Die Schwebelaryngoskopie und ihre praktische Verwertung.* (*Suspension laryngoscopy and its practical use.*) Berlin:
[20] Chevalier Jackson (1910). *J. Amer. med. Assoc.,* June 18. 2012.
[21] Chevalier Jackson (1958). *Brit. med. J.,* Aug. 30. 568.
[22] *J. Amer. med. Ass.* (1909), Sept. 25. 1011.
Holborn Surgical Instrument Company (1957). Catalogue.
[23] *Brit. med. J.* (1906), Nov. 24. 1482.
[24] E. Watson Williams (1932). *Lancet,* Mar. 12. 566.
[25] E. Fletcher Ingals (1909). *J. Amer. med. Ass.,* May 8. 1495.
[26] R. G. MacBeth and Freda Bannister (1944). *Lancet,* Nov. 18. 660.
[27] W. W. Mushin and L. Rendell-Baker (1953). *Principles of Thoracic Anaesthesia.* Oxford: Blackwell.
[28] Robert A. Miller (1941). *Anesthesiology.* Vol. 2. 318.
[29] N. A. Gillespie (1948). *Endotracheal Anaesthesia.* 2nd ed. University of Wisconsin Press.
[30] W. A. Cassels (1942). *Anesthesiology.* Vol. 3. 581.
[31] Sidney C. Wiggin (1944). *Anesthesiology.* Vol. 5. 61.
[32] R. R. Macintosh (1941). *Brit. med. J.,* Dec. 27. 914.
[33] R. R. Macintosh (1943). *Lancet,* Feb. 13. 205.
[34] R. R. Macintosh (1944). *Lancet,* Apr. 8.
[35] G. F. Gibberd and J. B. Blaikley (1935). *Lancet,* July 20. 138.
[36] Alan Moncrieff (1935). *Lancet,* Mar. 23. 669.
[37] N. A. Gillespie (1948). *Endotracheal Anaesthesia.* 2nd ed. University of Wisconsin Press.
[38] Robert A. Miller (1946). *Anesthesiology.* Vol. 7. 206.
[39] Phyllis F. L. Daplyn (1946). *Brit. med. J.,* July 27. 117.
[40] J. S. Lundy (1942). *Clinical Anesthesia.* Philadelphia: Saunders.
[41] James A. Bennett (1943). *Anesthesiology.* Vol. 4. 27.

[42] Arnold & Sons, London (1954). *Catalogue of Veterinary Instruments.*
[43] H. E. G. Boyle and G. E. Gask (1912). *Lancet,* Nov. 30. 1520.
[44] Robert E. Kelly (1912). *Brit. med. J.,* July 20. 113.
(1913). *Brit. med. J.,* Apr. 5. 720.
[45] Moses Salzer (1913). *J. Amer. med. Ass.,* Mar. 15. 826.
[46] C. A. Elsberg (1913). *Med. Ann.* Vol. 5.
[47] Willy Meyer (1909). *J. Amer. med. Ass.,* Dec. 11. 1984.
[48] Willy Meyer (1911). *Med. Rec. N.Y.,* June 17. 1079.
[49] Sterling Bunnell (1912). *J. Amer. med. Ass.,* Mar. 23. 836.
[50] H. Morriston Davies (1911). *Brit. med. J.,* July 8. 61.
[51] R. R. Macintosh and W. W. Mushin (1943). *Brit. med. J.,* Aug. 21. 234.
[52] John E. Grimm and Ralph T. Knight (1943). *Anesthesiology.* Vol. 4. 7.
[53] B. B. Lennon and E. A. Rovenstine (1939). *Curr. Res. Anesth.* Vol. 18. 218.
[54] J. S. Lundy (1942). *Clinical Anesthesia.* Philadelphia: Saunders.
[55] Mark I. Knapp (1896). *Med. Rec. N.Y.,* Aug. 29. 322.
[56] Mark I. Knapp (1898). *Med. Rec. N.Y.,* Feb. 26. 313.
[57] W. W. Mushin and L. Rendell-Baker (1953). *Principles of Thoracic Anaesthesia,* Fig. 170. Oxford: Blackwell.
[58] W. W. Mushin and L. Rendell-Baker (1953). *Principles of Thoracic Anaesthesia,* Fig. 169. Oxford: Blackwell.
[59] Philip Ayre (1937). *Lancet,* Mar. 6. 561.
[60] Frank Cole (1945). *Curr. Res. Anesth.* Vol. 24. 263.
[61] Edwards Surgical Supplies. Catalogue. (Not dated).
[62] R. A. Gordon and E. H. Ainslie (1945). *Anesthesiology.* Vol. 6. 359.
[63] John E. G. McGibbon (1940). *Lancet,* June 15. 1083.
[64] John E. G. McGibbon (1941). *Lancet,* July 26. 101.
[65] Holborn Surgical Instrument Co. (1957). Catalogue.

CHAPTER 8

COUNSEL FOR THE DEFENCE, or THE ACCUSED GIVES EVIDENCE

"It is of fundamental importance, that justice should not only be done, but should manifestly and undoubtedly be seen to be done."

—LORD HEWART, *Lord Chief Justice of England.*

EARLIER in these essays[1] I had some very hard things to say about Charles T. Jackson, Morton's competitor and rival in the discovery and use of ether. These criticisms were made in good faith, and on what I believed to be good evidence. But they were mostly the opinions of others—in other words, evidence for the prosecution. The time has now come to let Dr. Jackson conduct his own case and speak in his own defence.

I knew that he had written a book on anæsthesia,[2] but I hardly thought it would be possible to get hold of it in this country. But that invaluable service, the Library Interloan system, eventually got it for me from the University of Manchester, at the modest cost of three shillings for postage, so at long last we can let Jackson speak for himself and attempt to assess the value of his evidence.

In my previous remarks about him I made use of two expressions, which were perhaps a little too dogmatic, and which, in the light of Jackson's book, should be modified, though my general opinion remains unchanged. There is some foundation for these expressions, but perhaps they went a little too far. I said that there was "no evidence that he ever used ether at all, although he wrote a book about it," and that "he did no work on anæsthesia himself, either theoretical or practical."

Jackson's book was entitled *A Manual of Etherization.*[2] This is cutting it short, for the full title contained 61 words. It was published in Boston in 1861. No reason is given for the long delay of fifteen years which elapsed from the discovery to the date of publication. It contains, quite frankly, a considerable amount of personal propaganda. There are many references, mostly from the French, to his own great services in the matter, and at the end of the book is a page which is nothing less than a personal business advertisement. It reads, in the displayed capital letters and the fancy type which appealed so strongly to the nineteenth century printer:—

A

MANUAL OF ETHERIZATION:

CONTAINING DIRECTIONS FOR THE EMPLOYMENT OF

ETHER, CHLOROFORM, AND OTHER ANÆSTHETIC AGENTS,

BY INHALATION,

IN

SURGICAL OPERATIONS,

INTENDED FOR MILITARY AND NAVAL SURGEONS, AND ALL WHO MAY BE EXPOSED TO SURGICAL OPERATIONS; WITH INSTRUCTIONS FOR THE PREPARATION OF ETHER AND CHLOROFORM, AND FOR TESTING THEM FOR IMPURITIES.

COMPRISING, ALSO,

A BRIEF HISTORY OF THE DISCOVERY OF ANÆSTHESIA.

BY CHAS. T. JACKSON, M. D., F. G. S. F.,

Chevalier de la Légion d' Honneur; Caviliere dell Ordine dei S. S. Maurizio é Lazzaro; Ritter des Rothen Adler; Knight of the Turkish Order of the Medjidieh; Member of numerous Scientific and Medical Societies in Europe and America.

BOSTON:
PUBLISHED FOR THE AUTHOR BY J. B. MANSFIELD,
39 Court Street.
1861.

FIG. 12

A Manual of Etherization. Chas. T. Jackson. 1861. Boston: J. B. Mansfield. Title page.

Charles T. Jackson, M.D., State Assayer, Analytic and Consulting Chemist, Mineralogist and Geologist. House and Office, 32 Somerset Street, Boston.

It may also be admitted that much of the book is compiled from the experiences of other people—statistics from Bouisson[3] and Simpson, quotations from Flourens and others on the physiological effects of ether and so on. But this is no proof that it is a bad book. After all, even the best textbooks do not, as a rule, depend wholly upon the author's personal experience. That is the case today even in anæsthetic books written by anæsthetists. It was still more so in the days when anæsthetic books were written by others—generally by surgeons.

Jackson's book, for its date, contains a pretty complete and comprehensive account of anæsthesia as it was then practised. The chapters on the chemistry of the drugs and their manufacture, purification and testing, are particularly good, as might be expected in view of Jackson's primary profession as a chemist and scientist. He was a medical man, but did not practice as such.

In fairness to him it will be as well to give a summary of his book, reserving the right to comment on it when necessary. It is not easy to reduce 127 pages of print to a reasonable length without omitting anything of importance, but the attempt must be made.

It is dedicated to M. L. Élie de Beaumont, Perpetual Secretary of the Imperial Academy of Sciences and Member of the Senate of France. Jackson had sent accounts of the discovery to the Academy in the early days of the controversy. Then follow three pages of "European opinions on Etherization."

"L'année 1846 sera cèlébre (sic) dans l'histoire des sciences: elle a vu . . . un nouveau corps céleste, déterminé par la seule puissance du calcul . . . enfin un agent efficace contre la douleur liée aux opérations chirurgicales. . . . Les deux mondes ont eu leur part de gloire. . . . Leverrier a glorifié l'humanité, Jackson l'a servie."

"The year 1846 will be celebrated in the history of science: it has seen . . . a new celestial body, discovered by the sole power of the calculus . . . (and) at last an effective agent against the pain inseparable from surgical operations. . . . The two worlds have had their share of glory. . . . Leverrier has glorified humanity, Jackson has served it."

It may be noted, as a matter of interest, that this account is just as one-sided and biased as some of Jackson's own statements. It is quite true that Urbain Jean Joseph Leverrier (1811-1877) performed the amazing feat of deducing the existence of an unknown planet from some unexplained irregularities in the orbit of Uranus, which at that time was the outermost planet of the solar system. Moreover he calculated the actual position of the unknown with such accuracy—all on theoretical grounds—that the planet Neptune was found by Galle of Berlin on September 23rd, 1846, within one degree of its predicted position. That was an astounding feat of reasoning and pure mathematics. But Bouisson does not add, as in fairness he should have done, that John Couch Adams (1819-1892), a twenty-six year old Fellow of St. John's College, Cambridge, had done exactly the same thing at about the same time. He completed his calculations in September, 1845, and the Cambridge observatory began to search for the suspected planet in July, 1846. Professor Challis actually saw it on August 4th, but without identifying it, so its first official discovery was recorded on the Continent.

Jackson behaves in a somewhat similar way. He hardly mentions Morton except to refer to him in derogatory terms or to minimise his part in the work.

His next quotation is from Dupuytren:—"La douleur tue comme l'hemorrhagie." And then two more fragments from Bouisson:

"A painful operation which requires half an hour is full of real dangers. If it extends a longer time the danger is no longer doubtful." . . . "An operation exceedingly painful, if continued for some time without intermission, will cause death by exhaustion of the nervous powers."

Then Jackson stops quoting and begins to put forward his own case.

"Whatever removes the exhausting pains arising from the dread shock of the surgeon's knife adds greatly to the chances of the patient's recovery. Strongly impressed with this belief, for many years I sought for some method of preventing the pain of a surgical operation. . . ."

Then he describes some of the methods used by preceding generations in vain attempts to relieve pain. Opium was inefficient and dangerous, because its systemic effects were too great before it produced any real anæsthesia. Severe cold, as reported by Baron Larrey after the battle of Eylau, could be effective, but it had its own dangers, notably gangrene and pneumonia. Drunkenness had been successful in isolated cases, but was not suitable for routine use. Mesmerism had also worked well in some cases, but was unreliable. Trials of it in the Massachusetts General Hospital many years before were a complete failure.

"Protoxide of nitrogen has been supposed by some persons to be an anæsthetic agent." He mentions Davy's suggestion in 1800. But Davy said that the pains came back after inhalation and that the gas could cause increased irritability, which was confirmed by Beddoes; so Jackson argues:

"Thus it appears from the researches of the discoverer of Protoxide of Nitrogen himself, and from the experience of his medical instructor and employer, Dr. Beddoes, that Protoxide of Nitrogen, or exhilarating gas, has no anæsthetic properties."

This, of course, was quite contrary to what Davy actually said. He was so sure of its pain-relieving qualities that he recommended its use in surgery.

"By oft-repeated experiments, inhaling Protoxide of Nitrogen myself and by administering it to others in every possible way, by large and small orifices, I soon became fully satisfied that it possessed no anæsthetic properties."

It is not necessary to believe that Jackson was lying, but I cannot think that his experience of gas was as large as he makes out. It would not need many trials to find out that it did work sometimes, even with primitive and unreliable apparatus. Jackson goes on to say that he did not see Horace Wells's experiments but understood from others that he failed to render his subjects insensible to pain. He then mentions Hickman and his unsuccessful attempts with carbon dioxide.

Chapter 2 begins:

"Discouraged by the want of favorable results from my experiments with protoxide of nitrogen, which I administered in every conceivable manner, I did not wholly abandon the idea of ultimately finding something that would produce the effect which I was in search of. . . ." "I was familiar with the fact that stupor had been in several instances produced by inhalation of ether vapor; but that was regarded at the time, by all who reported the cases, as an exceedingly dangerous state. . . . Orfila . . . and other high toxicological authorities had classed ether among the narcotic poisons, and had given instances of death from its inhalation." . . . "I knew, also, that college boys and factory girls had inhaled ether with the utmost freedom, without any ill-effects upon their health. . . . In the year 1837 I discovered that ether vapor was superior to that of alcohol as a remedy for the strangling and toxical effects resulting from the inhalation of chlorine gas, and it was used for that purpose in my laboratory from that time forth. . . . Familiarity with the influence of ether vapor prepared me for the discovery of its anæsthetic effects. . . ."

The King of Prussia ordered Baron von Humboldt to investigate the ether controversy, and the Baron applied to the State Department of the United States for copies of the evidence. The King sent Jackson the order of the Red Eagle in 1857. Jackson reprints a copy of the letter which he sent to von Humboldt in 1851:

"in the winter of 1841-2 one of these large jars . . . filled with pure chlorine . . . overturned and broke, and in my endeavours to save the vessel, I accidentally got my lungs full of chlorine gas, which nearly suffocated me, so that my life was in imminent danger. I immediately had ether and ammonia brought, and alternatively inhaled them with great relief. The next morning my throat was severely inflamed and very painful. . . . I determined, therefore, to make a more thorough trial of ether vapor. . . . I had a large supply of perfectly pure washed sulphuric ether. . . . I took a bottle of that ether and a folded towel, and . . . placed my feet in another chair. . . . Soaking my towel in ether I placed it over my nose and mouth, so as to allow me to inhale the ether vapor mingled with air. . . . At first it made me cough, but soon that irritability ceased, and I noticed a sense of coolness followed by warmth. . . ."

Jackson then goes on to describe the symptoms of analgesia to the stage of unconsciousness in such minute and accurate detail as to convince me that the incident actually happened. The pain in his throat temporarily disappeared.

"Reflecting on these phenomena the idea flashed into my mind that I had made the discovery I had for so long a time been in quest of—a means of rendering the nerves of sensation temporarily insensible, so as to admit of the performance of a surgical operation on an individual without his suffering pain therefrom."

Jackson does not make clear his reasons why he considered ether to be a suitable anæsthetic for "the most severe surgical operations." After all, the pain in his throat came back again when the inhalation was discontinued—and this was the very argument that he had previously used in dismissing nitrous oxide as useless. Nor does he state, when he had at long last found the thing he had been looking for for so many years, the thing which would add so greatly to the chances of the patients' recovery, why he waited from the winter of 1841-2 until 1846 to bring it before the world. This is perhaps the weakest point in his whole case.

Perhaps he realised this, for he next gives a list of fifteen people (eight of them non-medical) to whom he had communicated his discovery, beginning with George Darricot, Esq., engineer, in the winter of 1841-42, including W. T. G. Morton, dentist, on September 30th, 1846 (No. 11

in chronological order) and ending with October, 1846, Dr. John C. Warren. There are three doctors and one dentist in the list before Morton. If Jackson really made the discovery, as he said, in the winter of 1841-2, and was really anxious to find a method of anæsthesia, as he claimed, why did he not succeed in interesting one of these four in it? Or, failing them, somebody else. Why did he wait five years, knowing that ether was the answer to the problem, before mentioning it to Morton, whom he always professed to be an ignoramus, a mere unskilled mechanic?

He does make some attempt to explain this curious inaction, but it is not very convincing. After saying that ether was used in the treatment of one of his assistants, Dr. Wm. F. Channing, for an accidental chlorine inhalation similar to Jackson's own, he states that he persuaded Joseph Peabody, another chemistry pupil of his, to take ether for two dental extractions, but Peabody's father showed him books on toxicology which stated that ether was extremely dangerous. He had also tried to persuade Dr. S. A. Bemis, a dentist, to use it. "I felt slighted by his not embracing my proposal at once."

Were these sporadic, feeble and abortive attempts the attitude one would expect from a well known scientist who had at last found the solution to the vitally important and world wide problem of pain, and knew that it was what he had been seeking for years? Hardly, I think. Reticence which was difficult enough to understand in a retiring and obscure country doctor like Crawford W. Long, becomes impossible to believe in a person of Jackson's reputation, pushful character and propensity to self-advertisement.

Jackson then states that in 1847/48/49, when working as U.S. geologist on Lake Superior, he frequently gave ether and chloroform to Indians and miners for small operations. One Indian, for extraction of a tooth, was kept under for four hours with a mixture of ether and chloroform "to convince the missionaries at l'Aunce station that a person could be kept in that condition long enough for any surgical operation." Well, of course, there is nothing improbable in all this, though four hours as a demonstration does seem to be overdoing it a bit. The chapter ends with two more French testimonials, one of which[4] runs: "It is very easy to see that the numerous competitors of Mr. Jackson have no right to his discovery, and that the honor is reserved for him exclusively."

Chapter 3 gives nine pages of details for making and purifying ether. The distillation, washing and separating processes are described in full, together with tests for purity. The danger of fire is stressed—the condenser must be in another room, separated from the fire under the still by an airtight wall. A Davy safety lamp must be used if light is required in the condensing room. Chapter 4 deals with chloroform, called C_2HCl_3, and describes its manufacture and testing for purity. These two chapters are good, for Jackson was on his own ground here, in the familiar surroundings of the chemical laboratory. He gives a list of

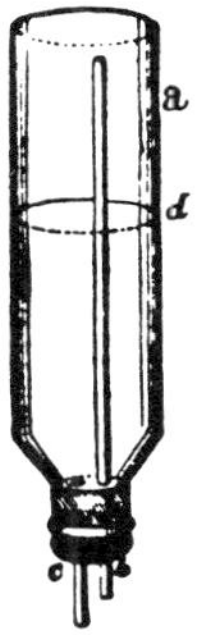

FIG. 13

A Manual of Etherization. Chas. T. Jackson. 1861. p. 32. Washing apparatus for ether. *a*, glass jar; *b*, air tube; *c*, tube for drawing off water first and then the ether; *d*, division line between the ether and the water.

A stopcock may be attached to the tube *c*, which may be made of metal. Lime water may be used instead of water if there is any acid in the ether.

Into the bottle, right end up, pour the ether, then add the water or lime water, shake up thoroughly. Cork it up. Invert it. Let it stand until the line of demarcation forms. Open tube *c* and let out the water. Hydrous ether with 1/36 its bulk of water remains. If dry ether is wanted it must be distilled off from powdered chloride of calcium.

twelve other substances used for anæsthesia: hydrochloric ether, acetic ether, nitrous ether, nitric ether, aldehyde, chloride of hydrocarbon, formomethyle, benzine, bisulphide of carbon, amylene, oil of turpentine and kerosolene. He claims to have tried Nos. 1, 5, 6, 9 and 12 on his own person, and to have given No. 9 to a pupil, but found it too powerful and too dangerous, producing well-marked asphyxia. Nitrous ether, he says, is a deadly poison.

The next chapter considers the introduction of etherization into surgical practice. He begins by quoting another prophecy which went wrong. Velpeau in 1839[5] said:

"Éviter la douleur dans les opérations est une chimère qu'il n'est pas permis de poursuivre aujourd'hui. Instrument tranchant et douleur, en médicine opératoire, sont deux mots qui ne se présentent point l'un sans l'autre à l'esprit des malades, et dont il faut nécessairement admettre l'association." (To avoid pain during operations is a chimera which it is not permissible to follow today. Cutting instrument and pain, in operative surgery, are two words which never present themselves one without the other to the minds of patients, and it is necessary to admit the connection."

But, Jackson goes on,

"it is proper for me to state, at once, that he was also one of the very first to adopt and defend my discovery of etherization. . . ."

"Having confided my discovery to twelve of my friends (p. 48), most of whom are gentlemen devoted to science, and some of them physicians and dentists, I considered it safe, so far as priority of discovery was concerned."

There is a discrepancy here. On p. 23 he gives a list of fifteen friends. According to this table, which is in chronological order (with one apparent misprint in No. 10) he had confided in ten people only before the date on which Morton first tried ether on Eben Frost. On that date the secret was given to Morton and two others—three in all. So, according to the date chosen, the number should have been ten or thirteen, not twelve.

Considering his discovery safe, Jackson continued:

"It was my intention to revisit Europe, and to bring out this discovery in the great hospitals of Paris, where I felt confident that I should be treated with courtesy and fairness; but I was at the time actively engaged in the Geological Survey . . . so that I had not a month that could be spared for a voyage to Europe. . . . Under these circumstances, I employed a dentist, a nominal medical pupil of mine, to make trial of my discovery, in dental surgery, which he consented to do, if I would take the entire responsibility."

Really Dr. Jackson was most unfortunate—at every turn he was thwarted. Either he was away from home, or he was too busy to leave home, or nobody told him about the operation—there was always some reason why he was never there when his great discovery was used.

On the 30th September Morton gave ether to Eben Frost and took out a tooth, without pain. In this case no reason is given why Jackson was not present. The presumption is that Morton's account was correct—that the case was an emergency, due to toothache, so he did the job entirely on his own initiative and responsibility. In Jackson's account—

"the tooth having been extracted by the dentist above named, who operated as directed by me. . . . The case was promptly reported to me the next morning." (Remote control again!) "I then engaged this dentist to go to Dr. John C. Warren and ask him to test the ether in a more severe case at the Hospital. The reason why I did not go in person was that I was at that time engaged in chemical work for others, which could not be left."

Perhaps as a result of his absence on this occasion:

"I was not informed when the trial of the ether was to be made at the Hospital, and it was done the next day, without notifying me that I might attend and witness the effects."

This would be Gilbert Abbott's case on October 16th, the famous first public demonstration, and again Jackson was not there.

But he saw Warren soon afterwards and states that Warren asked him to come to the hospital and give the ether himself, "as he did not like to have such a quackish fellow as Morton about the hospital." But, no, again Jackson had other engagements "but would fully instruct Morton and send him to administer the ether." This, from a person who had never even seen an anæsthetic given, with the exception of one personal trial upon himself, is distinctly good. Morton had at least used ether on Eben Frost, and, in public, upon Gilbert Abbott, in addition, as his son stated later, to 37 private cases for Dr. Bigelow.[6]

On Jackson's return from Maryland he found that he had missed yet another case. "I then . . . went with (Dr. Warren) to see an operation on a private patient at the Broomfield House, where a small tumor was removed from the thigh of a man, the Hospital house surgeon administering the ether." No date is given, but this must have been November 21st, for that was the date on which Jackson, by evidence from other sources, saw his first anæsthetic.[7] The nature of the operation also fits this case.

> "During the winter of 1846 . . . I continued to attend the most important surgical operations at the Massachusetts General Hospital, by invitation of Dr. John C. Warren, the chief surgeon, and at his request frequently gave advice and directions, so as to avoid accidents in etherizing patients. I have also frequently assisted my surgical friends by administering ether and chloroform."

This is a little misleading. It is all in one paragraph, but the reference to chloroform is not appropriate to the date, because chloroform was not then in use. The last sentence must refer to a year later, at the very least. Perhaps this was just a slip of the pen on Jackson's part. After all, the book was not published until fifteen years after the events described. Jackson does not explain why he was asked to give advice and directions about anæsthesia as early as the winter of 1846. Morton was the only man with any experience to speak of at that date.

A footnote in this chapter refers to Crawford W. Long's operations on March 30th and July 3rd, 1842, "but a few months after I made the discovery of anæsthesia." Now we know why Jackson had repeatedly mentioned the winter of 1841-42. Even Long had to take second place to himself. He (Long) also operated under ether on September 9th, 1843, and January 8th, 1845. In 1844 Dr. Smiley amputated the arm of a person who had inhaled ether from an ethereal solution of opium. But Dr. Smiley thought that the effect was due to the opium.

Jackson then "most earnestly protested" against the patent. "My name was most reluctantly, on my part, allowed to go into the petition, and only for the sake of securing my scientific rights as the discoverer. . . ."

Jackson wrote to the French Academy of Sciences on 13th November, 1846, but kept the letter back until the 1st December, as Morton's agent had requested. He claims that it was not until his letters were received that ether was given successfully in France and Europe. Details of many French operations are then given, taken from Comptes Rendus.

Chapter 6, on the administration of ether, gives pictures of three ether inhalers. Figure 2 on p. 79 is described as "The first form of Inhaler employed by me." Figure 3, on p. 80, is "The next inhaler proposed by me." These three inhalers, says Jackson, are the best available, but "I dispense with all inhalers, and employ the towel, handkerchief or sponge." Morton had come to this conclusion, and had said so publicly, fourteen years earlier,[8] so that Jackson's claim was not exactly original.

"In presenting the sponge, charged with ether . . . pour on only a little ether. . . . If signs of wild excitement begin . . . overpower the patient at once by a stronger dose of the ether. . . ." He then advises that another woman should be present if the patient is a woman, and also that "the person who administers the ether should be a medical man, that he may be able to judge of the symptoms exhibited by the patient."

Silence is recommended during induction. He then devotes nearly a page to the signs of anæsthesia.

"I taught one of my young men, who served as an assistant, to manage the administration of ether so that he could hold any patient safely in an insensible state for an hour or longer without the least danger to life. . . ."

Several pages of statistics follow, quoted from Bouisson and Simpson.

"The preparation which I directed for military use, was four measures of ether and one of pure chloroform, mixed. This was styled éther chloroformé, in the armies of the Crimea."

The uses of anæsthesia for the detection of malingering are then mentioned. No person under ether can be held responsible for his actions.

"An instance has also been alluded to . . . in which a dentist had a large glass inhaler dashed to pieces upon his head by a patient under the exciting effects of common alcoholic ether of commerce. The dentist was properly punished for administering an impure ether, not fit to be used. . . ."

Hard drinkers especially are excited by ether.

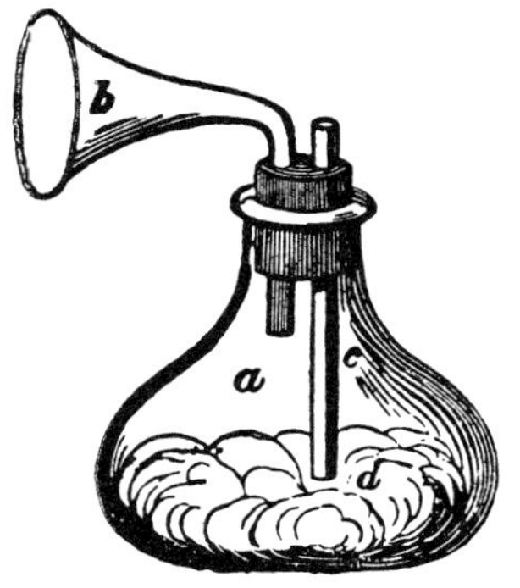

FIG. 14

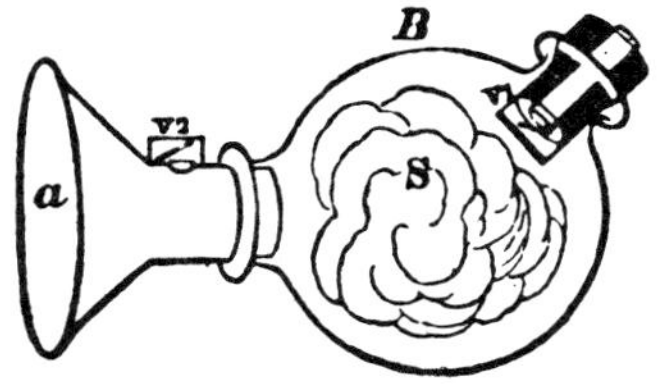

FIG. 15

FIG. 14

A Manual of Etherization. Chas. T. Jackson. 1861. p. 79. "At first I made use of a towel, folded into a cone, the interior of which was saturated with ether. . . . I also made use of sponges, placed in a large, short glass tube, or a funnel, saturated with ether. . . . Apparatus for inhaling having been called for, I proposed to make use of a large flask. . . . The first form of inhaler employed by me: *a*, glass flask, of three pints capacity; *b*, mouth-piece for inhalation of ether vapor; *c*, tube for admission of air, and for supplying the sponges with more ether; *d*, sponges, wet with ether. The air is drawn down the tube *c*, and over the sponges, wet with ether, which evaporates and mingles with the air, and is then drawn into the lungs through the tube and mouth-piece. A flap of buckskin, attached to the rim of the mouth-piece, makes the contact over the mouth secure. The air is inhaled and exhaled through the apparatus freely.

FIG. 15

A Manual of Etherization. Chas. T. Jackson. 1861. p. 80. "I also employed a globular glass receiver with a large neck, sufficient to cover the mouth, and a tubulure for the admission of air, the globe being filled with pieces of sponge saturated with ether. To a globe of this kind, Dr. A. A. Gould applied Mawes' syringe valves, so as to prevent the exhaled air from returning to the inhaler.

"Fig. 4 is the next inhaler proposed by me, which subsequently had valves affixed at the suggestion of Dr. A. A. Gould—this being the apparatus employed at the Massachusetts General Hospital. It was constructed by N. B. Chamberlain, of Boston. *a*, mouthpiece, with valve V2 for exhalation; B, glass globe; *a*, Common two-quart globular condenser, used by chemists, with a valve for the admission of air, V1. S, sponges wet with ether. The ether is renewed by taking out the valve seat V1, or by removal of the mouth-piece, and some delay is caused by this; it would therefore be advisable to have another tubulure at B, for injecting ether without the removal of the apparatus. Such a contrivance was added by M. Charriere of Paris."

Jackson claims that on one occasion at the hospital he found that the valve stuck and caused asphyxia. A probe to free it was used, instead of the bag of oxygen which he had taken with him.

Chapter 7. Most of the early failures were due to imperfect apparatus, inferior quality of ether or lack of skill. Still, some patients are difficult,

> "and a few whose constitutions have been so hardened by the habitual and excessive use of ardent spirits as to render them completely proof against both ether and chloroform." . . . "In one instance I gave a pound of ether and a quarter of a pound of chloroform to a stout young seaman, who had just before drank a stiff glass of brandy to brace him against the pain of a dental operation. This enormous dose of ether and chloroform, faithfully inhaled, had no effect upon him than to produce nausea and vomiting. His tooth was extracted, and gave him as much pain as usual in such cases. In another instance I administered a still larger dose of these two anæsthetic agents . . . to a hard drinker. . . . He could not be rendered insensible to pain."

This account of the enormous quantity of ether and chloroform used rings true to me. It is unusual, so unusual that I think Jackson must have met it personally. I have not come across any such report in any of the early books on anæsthesia, from which he might have quoted it. I personally have met one case—one in 16,000—which was nearly as immune as Jackson's cases, but not quite, for I could get him under as far as the first or second plane of the third stage, but no further. It was many years ago, long before the relaxant era, when relaxation could be secured only by deep anæsthesia. The patient was a male adult for a cholecystectomy. I used a pound of ether and *a pound of chloroform* in this extraordinary case, and even then he was never properly relaxed. The anæsthesia probably lasted about an hour, as the surgeon was considerably handicapped by abdominal rigidity and straining. I am no lover of chloroform and very rarely used it. Generally I could get adequate relaxation with ether or cyclopropane. But this case defeated me utterly.

I have seen one other case in which it was impossible to quieten the patient with cyclopropane—and heaven knows that is powerful enough. This was at the Radcliffe Infirmary at Oxford. A very well known American anæsthetist, a master of the art, was staying in Oxford and he had been given a free hand in the anæsthetic department for the time being as a matter of courtesy and as a tribute to his fame. He was one of the pioneers of cyclopropane, and this case occurred when he had had at least five years' experience of that gas. Never have I seen such a concentration of it administered as for that induction. It began in the ordinary way, with a reasonable percentage being given in the expectation of a smooth, quiet induction. But things were quite otherwise. There

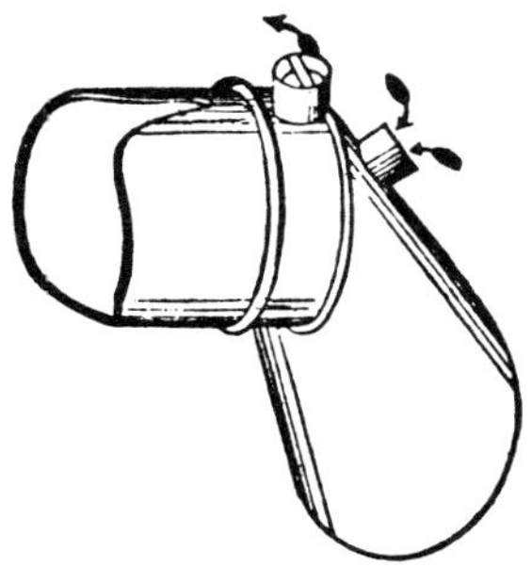

FIG. 16

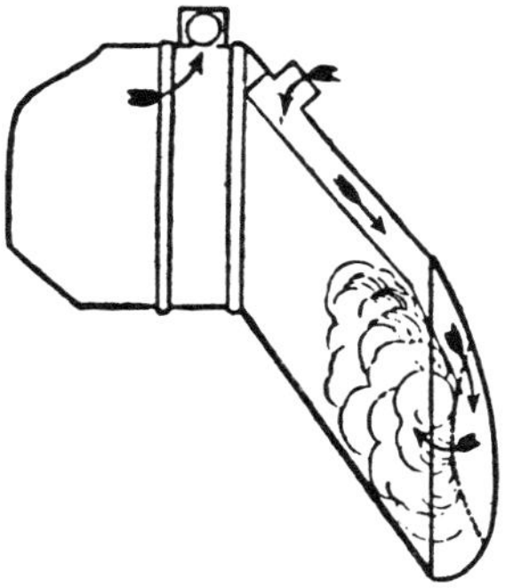

FIG. 17

FIGS. 16, 17

A Manual of Etherization. Chas. T. Jackson. Boston. 1861. p. 81. "Perspective and sectional views of Dr. L. Roper's inhaler, manufactured by Isaac S. Williams, at 256 Market Street, Philadelphia. This instrument is made of planished tinned iron and has a valve consisting of a loose marble, which is kept in place by a tin strap, and plays quite freely and easily. This valve at the orifice of the inhalation tube is the only one in the instrument, and is not likely to become in any way obstructed. The diameter of the inhaler is three inches; its length six inches. At the bottom of the inhaler is a grating, through which the inhaled air passes, and on which the sponge rests, so that when the sponge is wet with ether, the air passes freely through it and around it, and takes up the ether in vapor, which is inhaled from the mouth of the instrument, placed directly over the nose and mouth. This instrument is by far the best that has, thus far, been invented, and saves much of the ether, while it prevents it from dropping on the person, his clothes or the bed. It will also serve for the administration of chloroform, or for the mixture of ether and chloroform. The arrows indicate the course of the air and ether vapor, and the discharge of the exhaled air. It takes but a moment to renew the ether in this inhaler, it being poured into the opening, or a new sponge may be wet with ether, and be dropped into it, the exhausted one being removed. This instrument may easily be carried in the pocket, and it is not liable to injury, and is one with which an excited patient can do no harm."

was a struggling, fighting patient whom no amount of cyclopropane would apparently quieten. Up and up went the flowmeter until it was being given almost like nitrous oxide. Still the patient struggled, until he was finally subdued by an intravenous barbiturate.

I think, then, that Jackson, in his limited experience, did have the bad luck to come across two of these rare cases. He did at least know the ordinary doses of ether, for earlier in his book, on p. 87, he says:

"We judge wholly by the effect it has on the subject. The surgeon ought, however, to have at least a pint of ether on hand when he begins the process. Some require only an ounce, others four, six or eight ounces; refractory patients often inhale as much as a pint of ether."

French surgeons say that their patients are generally etherized in about five minutes. This, says Jackson, is ample evidence of temperate habits, and abuse of alcohol is very rare in France. Women are more readily affected than men—"Women are almost always temperate." Children are always facile subjects. Here Jackson, in his pre-occupation with the effects of alcohol, entirely fails to allow for bodily size and muscular strength. "There is also a marked difference in the susceptibility of different nations, apart from temperate or intemperate habits." I do not agree with Jackson here, but this is a mere personal opinion, based on an experience probably many times larger than his, and I am not putting it forward as evidence against him. According to my records I gave anæsthetics to patients of forty-nine different races and nations when I was a prisoner-of-war in Germany. They ranged from Sikhs to Chinese, from Germans to Red Indians, from Basutos to Maoris, and I never noticed any difference whatever, with one possible exception. Jews appeared to be more excitable than other races—but when one considers the precarious position of Jewish prisoners in Germany that is perhaps not surprising.

Chronic lung disease, according to our author, is no contra-indication to ether, but heart disease and a tendency to apoplexy are. His advice on induction is good. Do not stop if the patient struggles, but push the anæsthetic. Most patients can be got under in five minutes if the ether is given boldly and freely, but patients vary. It must be remembered that deep anæsthesia was not required or attempted at the time he wrote. This was not needed until the coming of abdominal surgery twenty years later. He claims that no fatal case has resulted from ether, so far as is known. European surgeons also think it is safer than chloroform, and he ventures the incorrect prophecy that "it is probable that, ere long, chloroform will be employed only to reinforce ether, and that mostly for Army purposes."

Chloroform was used by the French for 30,000 cases in the Crimea, with no deaths. The English experience was less fortunate. He points out that the English used chloroform, whereas the French employed it only in the form of Jackson's mixture of one part of chloroform to four of ether.

On the question of euthanasia, which J. C. Warren had mentioned with approval, Jackson claimed to have used it in a woman with peritonitis and puerperal convulsions. It was given to the stage of analgesia only, with much temporary relief and no loss of consciousness. He then quotes in full Warren's general conclusions on anæsthesia.

He stated that he had given ether in 8 cases for the treatment of insanity at the McLean Asylum, under Dr. Luther V. Bell. Maniacal and suicidal patients derived some benefit from it.

Chapter 8 consists largely of quotations from Flourens and others on the physiological effects of ether. Its veterinary use is then touched upon. Jackson states that he gave ether to a cougar or South American lion, which was very ferocious. It was confined to one end of its cage by a strong plank pushed through the bars so that it could not turn round. An ether-soaked sponge on the end of a rod was then passed in through the bars. When it appeared safe to do so the sponge was applied closely to its face and its claws were removed. They had apparently caused damage to many unwary people who had gone too close. One pound of ether was used, but much of it was wasted in the early stages of the induction.

Jackson then takes the opportunity for an attack on Morton. He points out that

"when quadrupeds are etherized their posterior extremities become paralyzed first. . . . Anyone who has seen a dog etherized will at once discover the falsehood of the assertion, extensively published by a pretender to the discovery of etherization (this was Morton), that an etherized dog leapt ten feet into the air and fell into a pond of water, for they will see that a dog cannot leap, nor even walk or stand, while under the influence of ether."

Discounting the ten feet as an exaggeration, Jackson forgets, or has not had enough experience to notice, that all sorts of violent movements can take place in the stage of excitement before the stage of muscular paralysis is reached. By his reasoning his own story of the patient who smashed the inhaler on the dentist's head could not possibly happen. But there is nothing in the least incredible in it.

He mentions Pirogoff's method of giving ether per rectum, and gives a list of 15 chloroform deaths quoted from Bouisson. Eight of these were French, one of them aptly described as "*mort foudroyante*"—death as from a thunderbolt. He then gives a list of 9 American cases, 8 of them certainly due to the chloroform, collected by himself. He gives, again from Bouisson, 5 deaths attributed to ether, at least 4 of which were probably due to other causes.

He finished, except for a table of contents, by giving a list of seventy-one books and pamphlets on anæsthesia "in the library of the author, and have been consulted in the preparation of this work."

Looked at from a purely anæsthetic point of view Jackson's book is not a bad one. It is much better than many of the early ones such as Warren's or Miller's. It is probably to a very large extent a compilation of other people's experience rather than his own, and by the time it was published there was a considerable amount of anæsthetic literature on which to draw. Jackson was an intelligent man and a scientist, even if he had a bee in his bonnet which was, perhaps, the beginnings of the insanity which finally overtook him, and he would have no difficulty in making an intelligible and comprehensive survey of a subject he really knew very little about. After all, most of the books on anæsthesia at that time were written by surgeons who knew little about, and had small interest in, anæsthetics. John Snow's books were the only genuine books on the market for very many years. But it is correct to say that Jackson's was one of the best of the 'ersatz' books.

It is notoriously difficult to draw conclusions as to personal experience from the internal evidence of a book written by someone who purports to have personal knowledge. A classical example of this is Daniel Defoe's *Journal of the Plague Year*. This is a description of the great plague of London in 1665 in such tragic and masterly detail that it is obviously the work of an eyewitness, of one who lived through that dreadful year. Defoe did live through it, and possibly in London, but he was only five years of age at the time! The book is in fact a *tour de force* of imaginative journalism, nothing more.

We have now heard the evidence for the defence and it is time for a judicial summing up.

The points in favour of Jackson are, firstly, that he had had a little personal experience of ether in the treatment of chlorine gassing. His description of ether analgesia is so good that I pass it as genuine. Second, he had had, at any rate, some practical experience of anæsthesia in the asylum, at Lake Superior, and with the two cases which needed enormous doses, not to mention the cougar. So I withdraw, or modify, the two statements which I made about him in an earlier essay. But his book, which no doubt contains all the evidence in his favour, in addition to quite a lot of propaganda, is not convincing and does not prove or even support his extensive claims.

Why did Jackson delay fifteen years before publishing it? Why did he exaggerate his experimental work with nitrous oxide? If it had been as extensive as he implied he could not possibly have dismissed it as having no anæsthetic properties. He claimed to discover the anæsthetic effects of ether in 1841-42, and to have realised its full implications at that date. Why did he wait until 1846 before making sure that somebody tried it? Why was there a discrepancy in his two accounts of the people to whom the great discovery was confided? Why did he eventually call upon Morton, whom he affects to despise, to use it? On no less than five occasions at the eventful beginning of a new era in surgery he could not be present when his discovery was used. Does this sound reasonable? If it was really Jackson's discovery why did Morton anæsthetise Eben Frost without Jackson being there, for Jackson said that Morton would only promise to try it if Jackson took the whole responsibility? Why did Morton anæsthetise Gilbert Abbott without Jackson's personal backing? Why did Jackson not see an anæsthetic used until November 21st, which was fifty-two days after Eben Frost's case and thirty-six days after Ether Day? Why was he asked to give advice and directions in 1846 when Morton was the only man with any practical experience? Was he not extremely fortunate in that his discovery date just anticipated Crawford W. Long who had by this time publicised his own claims in a modest way? If he knew so much about anæsthesia that he was asked to advise, why did he not give due weight to bodily size and muscular development in the patient as a factor in the ease and speed of induction, instead of attributing all difficulties to alcohol? If he knew so much, why did he say that the story of Morton's dog was impossible? Exaggerated, possibly, but certainly it was quite credible.

Another awkward point which requires an answer—and a good one—is the fact that Jackson sent a sealed packet to The Academy of Sciences in Paris. This was opened at the request of M. Élie de Beaumont, no doubt on Jackson's instructions, and found to contain two letters, the first one dated 13th November, 1846.[9]

At this date Jackson had not seen ether given in practice at all. Not until 21st November did he condescend to be present for the first time to see Morton, the 'ignoramus', give an anæsthetic for an operation. Jackson ignores this point, and begins,

"I am asking permission to communicate, by your intermediary, to the Academy of Sciences a discovery which I have made which I think important for the relief of suffering humanity, and of great value to the art of surgery.

"Five or six years ago I discovered the peculiar state of insensibility in which the nervous system is plunged by the inhalation of the vapour of pure sulphuric ether, in the first place by a trial and later at a time when I had a heavy cold caused by the inhalation of chlorine. Recently I devised a use for this fact by inducing a dentist of this city to administer the vapour of ether to persons from whom he was going to extract teeth. One noticed that these persons did not feel any pain during the operation, and that no inconvenience resulted from the administration of the ether vapour."

One also observes that Morton's name is not mentioned at all in this very one-sided account of the discovery. One further notices that Jackson's statement about absence of pain during operations was made eight days before he had first witnessed one.

"One can breathe this vapour very conveniently by immersing a large sponge in ether, putting it in a short conical tube or funnel, and inhaling the atmospheric air into the lungs through the sponge thus saturated in ether. The air can afterwards be breathed out by the nostrils, or better, one can fit valves to the tube or funnel in such a way that the breath does not pass out over the sponge, which would weaken the ether by the water vapour which it contains."

The extreme vagueness of the practical details is easily understood when one remembers that Jackson had never seen an anæsthetic given when he wrote this outrageous letter. He kept well out of the way at first in case the discovery was a flop, and all the responsibility, all the practical details, and the risk of failure or disaster were left to be borne by Morton, whose shoulders were fortunately broad enough to carry the load. The device of the sealed packet, which could be recalled or destroyed unopened in case of disaster, and Jackson's absence from the operating theatre for a whole five weeks after the first trial of his discovery, were all part of an ingenious heads-I-win-tails-you-lose scheme thought out by the twisted brain of Jackson himself.

"At the end of several minutes the patient falls into a very peculiar state of sleep and can be submitted to any surgical operation without feeling any pain; the pulse generally becomes a little more rapid and the eyes shine as if by the effect of a peculiar state of excitement: on recovery, at the end of a few minutes he tells you that he has slept and that he has dreamed. . . .

"If the dentist extracts teeth in the evening, it would be wise to have a Davy's safety lamp for the light, to avoid the danger of explosions caused by the ether vapour, which catches fire if a naked flame approaches the mouth."

This, perhaps, is one of Jackson's two really useful contributions to the discovery. Morton's experiment with ether in private, two weeks before his historic demonstration at the hospital, could so easily have ended in disaster. He gave ether to Eben Frost for the extraction of a tooth late in the evening, and an ordinary candle or lamp, held by Dr. G. G. Hayden, another dentist, was used for the necessary light. It was the merest fluke that the great discovery did not go up in flames, burnt to death at its very birth.

Jackson's second letter in the sealed packet was dated 1st December. The great discovery actually worked! There was no longer any doubt about it. Jackson had at last ventured to see it in use himself, and the moment had come for him to associate himself with it publicly. Let the seals be broken and the letter read, so that the great scientist should come into his own in place of the 'ignoramus'.

"The application of the vapour of ether has been used with great success at the Massachusetts General Hospital."

But this was not all. Another letter, dated 28th February, 1847, was received from Jackson. No secrecy about it this time. It was read at the session of the Academy held on 22nd March, 1847.[10] Still keeping up the pretence that he knew all about ether anæsthesia, Jackson stated that a case of prolonged insensibility had occurred. It will be remembered that Henry Bigelow had reported a case[11] in which anæsthesia was kept up for much longer than usual at that time—about twenty-five to thirty-five minutes. The patient only recovered after an hour. Quite probably this is the case which Jackson referred to. He then says:

"I propose to guard against such events by giving oxygen gas, which in a few moments, will bring back the colour of the blood and revive the patient. Everything should be ready in hospitals to treat such accidents. A copper gasometer and a bag of rubber-proofed fabric is sufficient to keep the gas ready for immediate use."

This again was another reasonable suggestion, but one which could not easily be adopted until oxygen was available commercially in cylinders about twenty-one years later. Making your own oxygen, collecting it and carrying it about in rubber bags was a very slow, complicated and cumbersome process.

One last question for Dr. Jackson to answer. Morton said that he studied in the office of Charles T. Jackson in the summer of 1844.[12] Presumably this was part of his M.D. course.

"About this time the wife and aunt of Dr. Jackson were under my treatment for dental purposes, and it was necessary to extract teeth in each case. . . ."

The quotation need not be continued here, as it will be dealt with in another essay. For our present purposes we need only ask, why, if Jackson considered Morton to be an ignoramus, did he entrust his wife and his aunt to him for dental treatment? Presumably at that time—in 1844—when the ether controversy had not yet arisen Jackson considered him to be a good dentist. There must have been other dentists in a city the size of Boston.

I fear that Dr. Jackson has quite a lot of awkward questions to answer before his case becomes at all convincing.

References

[1] Sykes, W. S. (1960). *Essays on the First Hundred Years of Anæsthesia.* Vol. I, p. 135. Edinburgh: Livingstone.

[2] Charles T. Jackson (1861). *A Manual of Etherization.* Boston: Mansfield.

[3] E. F. Bouisson (1850). *Traité Théorique et Pratique de la Méthode Anesthésique,* p. 3. Paris.

[4] M. H. Chambert (1848). *Effets Physiologiques et Thérapeutiques des Éthers,* p. 13. Paris.

[5] M. Velpeau (1839). *Médicine Opératoire.* Vol. 1, p. 32. Paris

[6] W. J. Morton (1911). *J. Amer. med. Ass.,* June 3. 1677.

[7] *Lancet* (1847), Apr. 3. 354.
Boston med. surg. J. (1847), May 26. 335.

[8] W. T. G. Morton (1847). *Lancet,* July 17. 80.

[9] *C. R. Acad. Sci.* (Paris) (1847). 74.

[10] *C. R. Acad. Sci.* (Paris) (1847). 492.

[11] Sykes, W. S. (1960). *Essays on the First Hundred Years of Anæsthesia.* Vol. I, p. 65. Edinburgh: Livingstone.

[12] Statements supported by evidence of Wm. T. G. Morton, M.D., on his claim to the discovery of the anæsthetic properties of ether submitted to the Honorable the Select Committee appointed by the Senate of the United States. 32nd Congress. 2nd Session. January 21. 1853. Washington (1853). P. 45.

CHAPTER 9

THE SECOND COMING OF THE NEWS TO SCOTLAND

Ether was used in Scotland for the first time on December 19th, 1846, by Dr. William Scott at the Dumfries and Galloway Royal Infirmary. This was the same day on which Dr. Boott and Mr. Robinson used it in London. This arrival of the news in Dumfries was discussed fully in a former Essay,[1] and need not be further considered here.

Very shortly afterwards the news came to Glasgow from an entirely different source. George Buchanan, who became the first Professor of Clinical Surgery at Glasgow University, gave some historical facts in his inaugural address on the 4th November, 1874,[2] twenty-eight years after the events he described:

"Two or three weeks after I was enrolled as a student of medicine, news came from across the Atlantic that Mr. Morton, a dentist in Boston, had extracted teeth without causing pain by making the patient inhale the vapour of sulphuric ether. The information was received in London on the 18th December, 1846, and on the 21st Mr. Liston, at University College Hospital, performed amputation of the thigh and avulsion of the toe-nail, the patients being quite unconscious of pain. The same night he wrote a note to my cousin, Mr. Buchanan, dentist in Glasgow, who had been a student of his, saying that as early information as to this property of ether might be serviceable to him, he placed the facts at his disposal. Immediately on the receipt of Mr. Liston's letter, Mr. Buchanan came to my father, who at that time was surgeon to the Infirmary, and having procured some ether, we began our experiment forthwith. My father and Mr. Buchanan were not successful, but with the assistance of another cousin well acquainted with chemical manipulation, Mr. G. S. Buchanan, I tried the experiment on myself. The ether was put in a glass globe with two necks, one of which I put in my mouth, while the air entered the flask by the other. In a few minutes I heard my cousin call out, 'He is slipping from the chair,' and then became unconscious. My father could not credit his eyes till he thrust his lancet under my nails till the blood flowed. Indeed, when I recovered consciousness I was inclined to disbelieve, till I saw the blood flowing from my nails. That is an old story now, but to me its memory comes back with all the vividness of a first year student. It is unnecessary to take up your time just now with any remarks on anæsthesia, but there is one point which I think has escaped the notice it deserves. In estimating the number of deaths which have happened under chloroform, there are various sources of error, one of which was forced on my attention in a remarkable way. When we consider the very small number of deaths from chloroform, and the large numbers of instantaneous or sudden deaths arising from what are called natural causes, the question arises: 'Have none of these chloroform deaths been really examples of deaths which would have happened independently of the administration of chloroform?' Three years ago, a patient with a small tumour of the lip was recommended to me by Professor Allen Thompson. The patient and his wife took lodgings in the vicinity of my house for my convenience. A day was fixed for the operation, but on the morning I received an urgent call to the country, so that the operation was postponed. The same evening the landlady called on me to tell me that her lodger had gone out for a walk in the forenoon and had not returned. Next morning I received the startling intelligence that my patient had fallen down dead in the street, at about midday, the very hour I had appointed for the operation. Had I, at that critical moment, been administering chloroform, I have no doubt that I myself would have attributed to it the death which happened as I have stated."

Liston wrote his letter on the evening of the 21st of December. It would arrive in Glasgow, possibly on the 22nd, or more likely, on the 23rd. The experiments appear to have been carried out the same day. If so, this would be four days after its first use at Dumfries.

There is only one other point which calls for comment. Buchanan is quite right when he says that a death under chloroform could be due to natural causes. The case he describes is presumptive evidence of that; but it is not an excuse that can often be used. Such a coincidence must be rare indeed, and it was extremely lucky for him that the operation had to be postponed.

References

[1] Sykes, W. S. (1960). *Essays on the First Hundred Years of Anæsthesia.* Vol. I, p. 50. Edinburgh: Livingstone.

[2] *Lancet.* (1874), Nov. 21. 722.

CHAPTER 10

CLASSICAL ARTICLES

Discovery of a new anæsthetic agent more efficient than Sulphuric Æther. By J. Y. Simpson, M.D., *Professor of Midwifery in the University of Edinburgh, Physician Accoucheur to Her Majesty in Scotland, etc.*[1]

At the first Winter Meeting of the Medico-Chirurgical Society of Edinburgh, held on the 10th of November last, I had an opportunity of directing the attention of the members to a new agent which I had been using for some time previously, for the purpose of producing insensibility to pain in surgical and obstetric practice.

This new anæsthetic agent is chloroform, chloroformyle, or perchloride of formyle.* Its composition is expressed by the chemical formula, C_2HCl_3. It can be procured by various processes, as by making milk of lime or an aqueous solution of caustic alkali act upon chloral; by distilling alcohol, pyroxylic spirit, or acetone with chloride of lime; by leading a stream of chlorine gas into a solution of caustic potass in spirit of wine, etc. The resulting chloroform obtained by these processes is a heavy, clear, transparent liquid, with a specific gravity as high as 1·480. It is not inflammable. It evaporates readily and boils at 141°. It possesses an agreeable, fragrant, fruit-like odour, and a saccharine pleasant taste.

As an inhaled anæsthetic agent it possesses, I believe, all the advantages of sulphuric æther, without its principal disadvantages:

1. A greatly less quantity of chloroform than of æther is requisite to produce the anæsthetic effect; usually from a hundred to a hundred and twenty drops of chloroform only, being sufficient, and with some patients much less. I have seen a strong person rendered completely insensible by six or seven inspirations of thirty drops only of the liquid.

2. Its action is much more rapid and complete, and generally more persistent. I have almost always seen from ten to twenty inspirations suffice; sometimes fewer. Hence the time of the surgeon is saved; and

*In making a variety of experiments upon the inhalation of different volatile chemical liquids, I have, in addition to perchloride of formyle, breathed chloride of hydrocarbon, acetone, nitrate of oxide of ethyle, benzin, the vapour of iodoform, etc. I may probably take another opportunity of describing the results. It is, perhaps, worthy of remark, that in performing his experiments upon inhalation, Sir Humphrey Davy confined his attention to the inspiration of gases, and does not seem to have breathed the vapour of any volatile liquids.

that preliminary stage of excitement, which pertains to all narcotizing agents, being curtailed or indeed practically abolished, the patient has not the same degree of tendency to exhilaration and talking.

3. Most of those who know from previous experience the sensations produced by æther-inhalation, and who have subsequently breathed the chloroform, have strongly declared the inhalation and influence of chloroform to be far more agreeable and pleasant than those of æther.

4. I believe that, considering the small quantity requisite, as compared with æther, the use of chloroform will be less expensive than that of æther, more especially as there is every prospect that the means of forming it may be simplified and cheapened.

5. Its perfume is not unpleasant, but the reverse; and the odour of it does not remain for any length of time obstinately attached to the clothes of the attendant, or exhaling in a disagreeable form from the lungs of the patient, as so generally happens with sulphuric æther.

6. Being required in much less quantity, it is much more portable and transmissible than sulphuric æther.

7. No special kind of inhaler or instrument is necessary for its exhibition. A little of the liquid diffused upon the interior of a hollow-shaped sponge, or a pocket-handkerchief, or a piece of linen or paper, and held over the mouth and nostrils, so as to be fully inhaled, generally suffices in about a minute or two to produce the desired effect.

I have had an opportunity of exhibiting chloroform with perfect success in various severe surgical operations (removal of tumours, of necrosed bone, amputations, &c., &c.), and in tooth-drawing,* opening abscesses, &c., &c.; for annulling the pain of dysmenorrhœa and of neuralgia; in two or three cases where I was using deep and otherwise very painful galvano-puncture for the treatment of ovarian dropsy; and

*A young dentist, who has himself had two teeth extracted lately, one under the influence of æther, and the other under the influence of chloroform, writes me the following statement of the results:—About six months ago I had an upper molar tooth extracted whilst under the influence of æther, by Mr. Imlach. The inhalation was continued for several minutes before I presented the usual appearance of complete ætherization. The tooth was then extracted; and although I did not feel the least pain, yet I was conscious of the operation being performed, and was quite aware when the crash took place. Some days ago I required another molar extracted on account of tooth-ache, and this operation was again performed by the same gentleman. I inhaled the vapour of chloroform, half a drachm being poured upon a handkerchief for that purpose, and held to my nose and mouth. Insensibility took place in a few seconds; but I was so completely *dead* this time, that I was not in the very slightest degree aware of anything that took place: the subsequent stupifying effects of the chloroform went off more rapidly than those of the æther; and I was perfectly well and able again for my work in a few minutes.

in removing a very large fibrous tumour from the posterior wall of the uterus by enucleation, &c.*

I have employed it also in obstetric practice with entire success. The lady to whom it was first exhibited during parturition, had been previously delivered in the country by perforation of the head of the infant, after a labour of three days' duration. In this, her second confinement, pains supervened a fortnight before the full time. Three hours and a half after they commenced, and ere the dilatation of the os uteri was completed, I placed her under the influence of the chloroform, by moistening, with half a teaspoonful of the liquid, a pocket-handkerchief, rolled up into a funnel-shape, and with the broad or open end of the funnel place over her mouth and nostrils. In consequence of the evaporation of the fluid, it was once more renewed in about ten or twelve minutes. The child was expelled in about twenty-five minutes after the inhalation was begun; the mother subsequently remained longer soporose than commonly happens after æther. The squalling of the child did not, as usual, rouse her, and some minutes elapsed after the placenta was expelled, and after the child was removed by the nurse into another room, before the patient awoke. She then turned round and observed to me that she had "enjoyed a very comfortable sleep, and indeed required it, as she was so tired,† but would now be more able for the work before her." I evaded entering into conversation with her, believing, as I do, that the most complete possible quietude forms one of the principal secrets for the successful employment of either æther or chloroform. In a little time she again remarked that she was afraid her "Sleep had stopped the pains." Shortly afterwards her infant was brought in by the nurse from the adjoining room, and it was a matter of no small difficulty to convince the astonished mother that the labour was entirely over, and that the child presented to her was really her "own living baby."

Perhaps I may be excused from adding, that since publishing on the subject of æther-inhalation in midwifery, seven or eight months ago,[2] and then for the first time directing the attention of the medical profession to its great use and importance in natural and morbid parturition, I have employed it, with few and rare exceptions, in every case of labour that I have attended, and with the most delightful results, and I have no doubt whatever that some years hence the practice will be general.

*I have now exhibited the chloroform to a large number of individuals, and in not one has the slightest bad effect of any kind resulted.

†In consequence of extreme anxiety at the unfortunate result of her previous confinement, she had slept little or none for one or two nights preceding the commencement of her present accouchement.

Obstetricians may oppose it, but I believe our patients themselves will force the use of it upon the profession.* I have never had the pleasure of watching over a series of better and more rapid recoveries, nor once witnessed any disagreeable result follow to either mother or child, whilst I have now seen an immense amount of maternal pain and agony saved by its employment; and I most conscientiously believe, that the proud mission of the physician is distinctly twofold—namely, to alleviate human suffering, as well as preserve human life.

In some remarks which I published in the *Monthly Journal of Medical Science,* for September, 1847, relative to the conditions for insuring successful ætherization in surgery, I took occasion to insist upon the three following leading points:

"*First,* the patient ought to be left, as far as possible, in a state of absolute quietude and freedom from mental excitement, both during the induction of ætherization and during his recovery from it. All talking and all questioning should be strictly prohibited. In this way any tendency to excitement is eschewed, and the proper effect of the æther-inhalation more speedily and certainly induced. *Secondly,* with the same view, the primary stage of exhilaration should be entirely avoided, or at least reduced to the shortest possible limit, by impregnating the respired air as fully with the æther-vapour as the patient can bear, and by allowing it to pass into the lungs both by the mouth and nostrils, so as rapidly and at once to induce its complete and anæsthetic effect, . . . a very common but certainly a very unpardonable error being to exhibit an imperfect and exciting, instead of a perfect and narcotizing, dose of the vapour. Many of the alleged failures and misadventures are doubtless entirely attributable to the neglect of this simple rule, not the principle of ætherization, but the mode of putting it in practice being altogether to blame. But, *thirdly,* whatever means or mode of ætherization is adopted, the most important of the conditions required for procuring a satisfactory and successful result from its employment in surgery, consists in obstinately determining to avoid the commencement of the operation itself, and never venturing to apply the knife until the patient is under the full influence of the æther-vapour, and *thoroughly and indubitably* soporized by it."

In fulfilling all these indications, the employment of chloroform evidently offers great and decided advantages in rapidity, facility, and efficiency over the employment of æther. When used for surgical purposes, I would advise it to be given upon a handkerchief, gathered up into a cup-like form in the hand of the exhibitor, and the open end of the cup

*I am told that the London physicians, with two or three exceptions only, have never yet employed æther-inhalation in midwifery practice. Three weeks ago I was informed in a letter from Professor Montgomery, of Dublin, that he believed that in that city, up to that date, it had not been used in a single case of labour.

placed over the nose and the mouth of the patient; for the first inspiration or two it should be held at the distance of half an inch or so from the face, and then more and more closely applied to it. To ensure a full and perfect anæsthetic effect—more especially when the operation is to be severe—a teaspoonful or two of the chloroform should at once be placed upon the hollow of the handkerchief, and immediately held to the face of the patient. Generally a state of snoring sleep very speedily supervenes, and when it does so, it is a perfect test of the superinduction of complete insensibility. But many patients are perfectly anæsthetic without this symptom.

As illustrations of the influence of this new anæsthetic agent, I will select and append notes of two operations performed with it on Friday last by Professor Miller, the first in the Royal Infirmary,* the other in private practice. The notes and remarks are in Mr. Miller's own words.

Case 1.—"A boy, four or five years old, with necrosis of one of the bones of the forearm. Could speak nothing but Gaelic. No means, consequently, of explaining to him what he was required to do. On holding a handkerchief, on which some chloroform had been sprinkled, to his face, he became frightened, and wrestled to be away. He was held gently, however, by Dr. Simpson, and obliged to inhale. After a few inspirations he ceased to cry or move, and fell into a sound snoring sleep. A deep incision was now made down to the diseased bone; and by the use of the forceps, nearly the whole of the radius, in the state of sequestrum, was extracted. During this operation, and the subsequent examination of the wound by the finger, not the slightest evidence of the suffering of pain was given. He still slept on soundly, and was carried back to his ward in that state. Half an hour afterwards he was found in bed, like a child newly awakened from a refreshing sleep, with a clear, merry eye and placid expression of countenance, wholly unlike what is found to obtain after ordinary etherization. On being questioned by a Gaelic interpreter (who was found among the students) he stated that he had never felt any pain, and that he felt none now. On being shown his wounded arm, he looked much surprised, but neither cried nor otherwise expressed the slightest alarm."

Case 2.—"A young lady wished to have a tumour (encysted) dissected out from beneath the angle of the jaw. The chloroform was used in small quantity, sprinkled upon a common operation sponge. In considerably less than a minute she was sound asleep, sitting easily in a chair, with her eyes shut, and with her ordinary expression of countenance. The tumour was extirpated, and a stitch inserted, without any pain having been either shown or felt.

*Professor Dumas, of Paris, Mr. Milne Edwards, Dr. Christison, Sir George Ballingall, and a large collection of professional gentlemen and students witnessed this operation, and two others performed with similar success, by Professor Miller and Dr. Duncan.

Her sensations, throughout, as she subsequently stated, had been of the most pleasing nature; and her manageableness during the operation was as perfect as if she had been a wax doll or a lay figure.

"No sickness, vomiting, headache, salivation, uneasiness of chest, in either of the cases. Once or twice a tickling cough took place in the first breathings.

"My assistant, Dr. Duncan, who exhibited the chloroform to this last patient, informs me that about a drachm of the liquid was used."

Edinburgh, November 15, 1847.

This was published in the *Lancet* (1847, Nov. 20. 549), and also in the *Provincial Medical and Surgical Journal* (1847, Dec. 1. 656).

Chloroform came into use very quickly. Simpson's first trial of it was on November 4th, his first announcement on November 10th. Dr. W. S. Wyman of Kettering reported an amputation under chloroform on November 27th. W. T. G. Morton had used it in Boston, Mass., before December 29th.

There are one or two comments to make on this very interesting and classical article. Simpson opened by referring to the "new agent which I had been using for some time." This, while strictly true, gives the impression of a length of experience which did not really exist at all. Few people would deduce from it the fact that he had only used chloroform for six days at the time of his first announcement.

In the second paragraph the formula is as Simpson gave it (C_2HCl_3). It is not a misprint on my part for $CHCl_3$.

Later he says, "I have now exhibited the chloroform to a large number of individuals." What this means is anybody's guess.

Dr. Matthews Duncan is just mentioned as giving the chloroform in one of the two cases described in the article. The fact that he took an equal part with Simpson in the preliminary personal trials on themselves is not mentioned at all. More surprising still, David Waldie, to whom Simpson owed the whole idea, is ignored completely, which seems hardly fair.

The preparation of Chloroform. By J. Y. Simpson.[3]

We have been favoured by Professor Simpson with the subjoined remarks on the preparation of Chloroform:

"I have seen different instances reported in the English and French Journals of patients requiring to inhale chloroform for five, ten, or even twenty minutes, before they came under its influence. In all such cases, the chloroform used must have been of a most inferior quality. I have generally seen patients affected in about a minute; they rarely resist it for above two minutes; and never, or almost never, above three. The chloroform which I have mostly used, is that manufactured by Messrs. Duncan, Flockhart, and Co., chemists, Edinburgh. It is made according to the following formula of Dumas:—

"R. Chloride of lime in powder,	lb. IV
Water,	lb. XII
Rectified Spirit,	f. oz. XII

"Mix in a capacious retort or still, and distil as long as a dense liquid, which sinks in the water with which it comes over, is produced.

"The product obtained by the above process, is rectified by agitating it with several portions of strong sulphuric acid, and afterwards distilling it from carbonate of baryta. Messrs. Duncan and Co. inform me, that they always distil it a *third* time from lime, and that they believe it would be impossible for them to furnish it perfectly pure without this. Latterly, they have made and sent out from 60 to 80 oz. per diem (2s. per oz.), manufactured by this process. In the observations which I previously published, I inadvertently omitted to state and insist upon the purifying part of the process.

"Of several specimens I bought in Glasgow, only *one* was of the proper strength and purity. I bought a specimen yesterday in an Edinburgh shop, sp. gr., only 1·130 instead of 1·480. There was little or no chloroform in it."

Dr. Simpson believes that all the reputed failures and misadventures are attributable to two causes: viz., (1) using an impure and imperfect variety of chloroform; and (2) not giving it in sufficiently large and rapid doses.

References

[1] *Prov. med. surg. J.* (1847), Dec. 1. 656.
Lancet (1847), Nov. 20. 549.
[2] See *Monthly Journal of Medical Science,* for Feb., p. 639; for March, p. 718, and 721, etc.
[3] *Prov. med. surg. J.* (1847), Dec. 29. 698.

CHAPTER II

DE PROFUNDIS

WHAT really possessed Horace Wells that he had such an unhappy and unsuccessful life and such a tragic death? As I see it, he was a man who was easily depressed and discouraged, too easily led and influenced by others; for after one partial public failure he completely abandoned his attempts to publicise nitrous oxide anæsthesia, which had already been satisfactory in his hands in a number of cases. We know that he was irresolute, wayward and volatile, for he kept abandoning his dental practice in order to make a living in strange and unusual ways, such as buying pictures in Paris to sell in the United States, and other queer ventures.

He was in fact the exact opposite of the phlegmatic Morton, who fought tooth and nail for his discovery against the persistent encroachments of Jackson; the exact antithesis of the rock-like Simpson, who thrived on controversy and dearly loved a fight. Only death itself silenced Simpson.

The facile way in which Wells helped his friend in the atrocious business of vitriol throwing shows that he was becoming more and more unbalanced as his short life drew to its close. In fact his last sane act was his realisation of his own degradation, which made him commit suicide to avoid disgrace to his family and to forestall the frank insanity which was engulfing him.

The last letters he wrote in the prison cell are pathetic in the extreme. In May, 1848, the case was reported:[1]

"Dr. Wells, the discoverer of the anæsthetic properties of æther (sic), having been placed in confinement on a charge of vitriol throwing, committed suicide by cutting the femoral artery of the left thigh with a razor. Previously to the fatal act, he inhaled some chloroform to produce some insensibility to pain. When discovered he was quite dead, and the cell in which he was confined was a pool of blood. On the floor were scattered several sheets of paper, on which the unfortunate man had written a history of the vitriol-throwing, the use and effects of chloroform, and the causes that led to his depriving himself of life. In one letter he says he became acquainted with a young man who frequented his office, as a dentist, that his friend called and said he would thank him (Dr. Wells) for some vitriolic acid, with which to pay back a loose female, who injured his (the friend's) dress—that he complied with the request of the young man, and that they prepared a phial to squirt the acid, by making a groove in the cork stopper thereof. The letter goes on to say, that they then sallied out into Broadway—that they met the female, on whose person vengeance was to be doled out—and that his acquaintance did so avenge the former injury.

"The friend then proposed that they should 'continue the sport', to which he gave a direct negative. They then parted, Dr. Wells going home. Afterwards he explains how he was accustomed to the use of chloroform, which he inhaled over and over again to produce the sensation of exhilaration. Two evenings after the one above mentioned, he used the chloroform, and in a moment of delirium he seized the phial of vitriol which was on the mantel, and rushing out into the street, commenced throwing it on the persons of the females who walked Broadway.

"The following is the conclusion of his statement in his own words:—'I lost all consciousness before I removed the inhaler from my mouth. How long it remained there I do not know, but on coming out of the stupor I was exhilarated beyond measure, exceeding anything I had ever before experienced, and seeing the phial of acid, I seized it and rushed into the street and threw it at two females. I may have thrust it at others, but I have no recollection further than this. The excitement did not leave me for some time after my arrest.' He says he did not so much care to free himself from blame by this communication, as to give to the world the real facts in connection with the fatal circumstances. The reason he gives for the crime on his own person which he was about to commit is, that he abominated the idea of doing mischief, and that he felt that his character was irrecoverably gone. In speaking of his wife and child, he says most feelingly, 'Oh, my God, protect them. I cannot proceed, my hand is too unsteady, and my whole frame is convulsed in agony. My brain is on fire'."

Sunday, 7 o'clock, p.m.

"I again take up my pen to finish what I have to say. Great God, has it come to this? Is it not all a dream? Before 12 to-night to pay the debt of Nature; yes, if I were free to go tomorrow I could not live and be called a villain. God knows I am not one. Oh, my dear mother, brother and sister, what can I say to you? My anguish will only allow me to bid you farewell. I die this night believing that God, who knoweth all hearts, will forgive the dreadful act. I shall spend my remaining time in prayer. Oh, what misery I shall bring on all my near relatives, and what still more distresses me is the fact that my name is familiar to the whole scientific world as being connected with an important discovery. And now, while I am scarcely able to hold my pen, I must to all say farewell! My God, forgive me! Oh, my dear wife and child, whom I leave destitute of the means of support, I would still live and work for you, but I cannot. Did I live I should become a maniac. The instrument of my destruction was obtained when the officer who had me in charge permitted me to go to my room yesterday. Horace Wells."

"To the Editors.—My last request to Editors is that they will, while commenting on this unhappy affair, think of my poor wife and child, also my mother, brother and sister, all of whom are amongst the most respectable members of society.

"To my dear wife.—I feel that I am fast becoming a deranged man, or I would desist from this act. I can't live and keep my reason, and on this account God will forgive the deed. I can say no more.

"To Mr. Dwyer, Western Hotel, Courtlandt Street.—

"Dear Sir,—When you receive this I shall be no more. I wish you would take my watch and present it to my dear wife, together with the trifle I have already given you. Please to attend to my burial, and let me be interred here in the most secret manner possible. I wish you and Mr. Barber would go immediately and reveal this misfortune to my wife in the most unobjectional manner possible, and attend to the business which we spoke of this morning, when you little thought of this occurrence.

Horace Wells.

Messrs. Dwyer and Barber, Western Hotel."

The deceased, as it is supposed, previously to committing the rash act, saturated a new silk handkerchief with the chloroform, and placed it to his mouth, where it was found tied by another silk handkerchief round his head. He was about 35 years of age. (This is not quite correct. To be exact he was thirty-three.)

The foregoing particulars relative to this extraordinary case are extracted from an American paper. We give the letters entire as exhibiting the state of mind of the writer at the time or immediately before the committal of the fatal act.

During a trip to Edinburgh to photograph Simpson's grave, we saw in Holyroodhouse a most pathetic letter written by Mary Queen of Scots on the eve of her execution. It was the most interesting thing in the Palace. She had been in prison for many years with her life dependent on the changeable whims of Queen Elizabeth; she was due to die in a few hours, no doubt, in her opinion, wrongly and unjustly. Pathetic and intensely moving it was, but Mary at least had the consolation of a clear conscience to lighten her burden.

Wells's state of mind when he wrote his last letters must have been far, far worse. His conscience was not clear. He was horrified by his crime and had remorse added to the darkness and despair of those last hours.

Reference

[1] *Brit. med. J.* (1848), May 31. 305.

CHAPTER 12

MR. JAMES MOORE GIVES AN ANÆSTHETIC FOR MR. JOHN HUNTER IN THE EIGHTEENTH CENTURY

IN Volume I of these Essays I illustrated Moore's nerve compression apparatus,[1] with a plate photographed from a book on surgery published in 1796. My main reason for showing this obsolete and not very efficient instrument was that I had often heard of it, but had never seen it illustrated in any modern book; but I was quite unable to find any description or account of it. Since that time I have found Moore's description, not in the original but quoted by Dr. J. Y. Simpson in 1848.[2] Simpson (he was not yet Sir James. He became a baronet in 1866) was rather fond of medical archæology. Amongst other subjects he wrote on the medical services attached to the Roman Legions.

Apparently Moore wrote a thirty-page pamphlet, which I have not been able to trace, entitled *A method of preventing or diminishing pain in several operations of Surgery*. By James Moore, Member of the Surgeons' Company, London. He then enlisted the aid of a very well-known surgeon in trying out his idea; one who above all others was constantly in search of something new.

"I communicated the experiments I had made and all my ideas on the subject to Mr. Hunter, who was so obliging as immediately to offer me an opportunity of trying out the effect of my compressor at St. George's Hospital, on a man whose leg he was to take off below the knee within a few days. I went to the hospital the day before the operation to try the instrument. The patient had lost all his toes, and had a large ulcer on his foot. This was so much inflamed and so irritable that dressing it in the gentlest manner gave him acute pain. I applied the instrument (which was rather like a curved carpenter's clamp with a screw adjustment); after the compression had been continued for about half an hour, his limb became so insensible that rubbing pretty smartly with the finger upon the ulcer gave no pain. Next morning, the patient being carried into the operation room, I began the compression of the nerves at a quarter before eleven o'clock. The numbness of the limb followed at the usual time. At a quarter before twelve I gave him one grain of opium to diminish the smarting of the wound after the operation, when the compression should be taken off. A few minutes after twelve the tourniquet was applied, and the amputation performed by Mr. Hunter, at the usual place below the knee.

"At the circular incision through the skin, the patient did not cry out, change a muscle of his face, or show any symptoms of pain. At the subsequent parts of the operation, particularly during the sawing of the bones, he showed signs of uneasiness in his countenance, but did not cry out. As it was thought necessary to take up no less than five arteries, the operation lasted a longer time than usual, and towards the end he grew faintish, and desired to have some water, and afterwards asked if they were nearly done. When the operation seemed to be over, and the bleeding stopt, the tourniquet was relaxed, and I also removed the compressor; but a small vessel bleeding unexpectedly, it was thought necessary to tie it also. Here the patient showed very strong marks of pain, and afterwards declared that tying this last vessel gave him much more pain than all the others, although the great nerves had been included in the ligatures. When he was put to bed the wound smarted as is usual after amputations. The compressor being now entirely removed this was to be expected. But some time after, being questioned concerning the pain he had suffered during the operation, he declared that he had felt hardly any, except, as he himself expressed it, at the rasping of the bones, which he added, had shaken his whole limb. This seems a little extraordinary, as sawing the bones is usually the least painful part of amputations. . . . This trial had all the success I expected; there was evidently a most remarkable diminution of pain, particularly during the first incisions through the skin and muscles, which are generally by far the most severe parts of the operation, and I am convinced that what pain the patient felt was chiefly owing to some small branches of the lumbar nerves which extend below the knee, and were not compressed."

This is a sober, factual account which carries conviction. It really does seem that the nerve compressor reduced the amount of pain considerably. The one grain dose of opium could not have had much effect in this way; the patient was normal in his sensitivity to pain, as proved by the ligature of a vessel after the compressor was removed.

It is rather extraordinary that, with no other means of anæsthesia at their disposal, the surgeons of that day did not take up the idea and use it frequently; but little more was ever heard of it. The date of the trial is not given; but it must have been between 9th December, 1768 and 1793, when Hunter was surgeon to St. George's Hospital. He died in office on October 16th, 1793.

References

[1] Sykes, W. S. (1960). *Essays on the First Hundred Years of Anæsthesia.* Vol. I, Plate IX. Edinburgh: Livingstone.

[2] *Prov. med. surg. J.* (1848), July 12. 365. (This was later renamed *Brit. med. J.*).

CHAPTER 13

PROPHECIES THAT WENT WRONG

"... but whether there be prophecies, they shall fail."
1 CORINTHIANS 13. 8.

SIR JOHN ERIC ERICHSEN, Bart., was born on July 19th, 1818. He qualified in 1839 and became surgeon to University College Hospital. He was one of the best known operators in London and wrote a surgical textbook which was looked upon as a work of great authority. He died on September 23rd, 1896. In 1873 he gave an introductory address to the new students at the beginning of the academic year. He stated that the knife could not always have fresh fields to conquer—that the limit had nearly, if not quite, been reached. "... if we reflect on the great achievements of modern operative surgery. Very little remains for the boldest to devise, or the most dexterous to perform."[1]

Many years later Sir St. Clair Thomson, who had been house surgeon to Lister in 1883, recalled this incident.[2] He said that at the time when Erichsen spoke his mortality from amputations was 25 per cent. which he considered "a very satisfactory result." He went on to prophesy, according to Thomson, that "the abdomen, the chest and the brain would be forever shut from the intrusion of the wise and humane surgeon."

The important point to notice here is the date on which Erichsen made these egregrious remarks—1873. Six years before Lister had published his first paper on his antiseptic method, and surgery had just begun. If Erichsen had said what he did say twenty years before, or even ten, there would have been some excuse. But he chose the one moment in all history when he should have kept his mouth shut. It is true that Lister himself never opened the abdomen, but this was not because of want of faith in his method. Four years after Erichsen's rash prophecy Lister opened the knee joint and wired the patella for the first time, which to other surgeons was just as dangerous and equally unjustifiable. Abdominal surgery was a field which Lister left to the younger surgeons to explore. He himself had quite enough to do in improving and perfecting the technique and details of his method. But a prophet hath no honour in his own country. Lister's principles were accepted and adopted far and wide in other countries before the London surgeons would condescend to try them. One of his great disappointments, when he left Scotland and went to London, was the fact that his class of students dwindled from several hundred to a mere dozen or so.

Velpeau, the famous French surgeon,[3] had made an almost equally rash forecast earlier in the century. It was not quite so bad, for at least he had the excuse that he spoke before there was any indication whatever that his words were soon to be proved wrong. Erichsen, on the other hand, stuck his neck out when the beginning of a new era was already in progress—for those who had eyes to see.

"Éviter la douleur dans les opérations est une chimère qu'il n'est pas permis de poursuivre aujourd'hui. Instrument tranchant et douleur, en médicine opératoire, sont deux mots qui ne se présentent point l'un sans l'autre à l'esprit des malades, et dont il faut nécessairement admettre l'association."

"To avoid pain during operations is a chimera which it is not permissible to follow today. Cutting instrument and pain, in operative surgery, are two words which never present themselves one without the other to the minds of patients, and it is necessary to admit the connection."

This was published a mere seven years before Ether Day. Even after this event, when anæsthesia was a *fait accompli*, Velpeau took a lot of convincing.[4] He said in 1847:

"Now is it necessary to take literally all the marvels which are uttered on this subject in the practical journals? No, without doubt. Here are the results of experience up to the present. One of my patients, a strong and robust man, who was to have an amputation of a finger, did not lose consciousness at all, and remained completely refractory to the action of the ether vapour. Another, at the end of ten minutes, was overtaken by a sort of drunkenness, with loquacity, with a peculiar blustering attitude, but was not at all prevented from feeling acutely the little operation which I performed on him. A young American became motionless at the end of three minutes and allowed the extraction without showing any sign of pain."

The next sentence is obscure and rather beyond my French, but seems to imply that he actually felt pain but could not move. "Three other persons inspired the ether vapour during five, eight and ten minutes without results. . . ."

M. Velpeau's argument is quite simple, and quite stupid. He couldn't do it properly at the first attempts—therefore it was impossible. Not for one moment did it occur to his mind that there might be anything to learn about anæsthesia.

Charles T. Jackson, the Boston analytical chemist and geologist, said in his book:[5] "It is probable that, ere long, chloroform will be employed only to reinforce ether, and that mostly for Army purposes."

This was a pretty inaccurate forecast. But Jackson knew very little about ether. His book was really a piece of personal propaganda, disguised as a textbook, but written to support his claim to be the originator.

Ranyard West, who did much work on curare in the 1930s, was very hampered by the extremely variable composition of his raw material. No two specimens were alike, so his results fluctuated wildly. This made his writings somewhat confused and difficult to follow. He did, however, come to a definite conclusion in 1935[6] that "I think the therapeutic uses of curarine will remain very limited." A short seven years later Griffith of Montreal brought it into general use.

G. P. Pitkin[7] ends a long and enthusiastic article on spinocain anæsthesia with the words "Permit me to foretell that, within ten years, possibly less, local, conduction, or spinal anæsthesia will be the anæsthetic procedure of choice." He was not the first to let his enthusiam outrun his discretion on this subject. Twenty years before—in 1909—Jonnesco of Bucharest advocated total or general spinal anæsthesia for everything, including skull and facial operations.[8] He said, after 400 cases, "General spinal anæsthesia is absolutely safe," and, "I am firmly convinced that general spinal analgesia will be the analgesic method of the future."

Thomas Nunneley, of Leeds, is mentioned elsewhere in these essays as an ardent recipient of the news of general anæsthesia and as a zealous seeker after new ideas. (Twenty years later he reversed his attitude completely and would not accept the idea of clean surgery at any price.)

He made many astonishing statements as a result of his experiments with different anæsthetic substances. Although these trials reached the respectable total of 363, he tested so many substances—well over thirty of them—that many of them were only tried a few times.[9]

"Though olefiant gas (ethylene) is an anæsthetic . . . it is not one of those which are likely to be used in practice." It must be remembered that he had no oxygen readily available, and that his experimental animals were tested in a somewhat crude way by being put into a jar filled with the vapour or gas being tested. So the factors of anoxæmia and carbon dioxide accumulation both came into play in a capricious and variable manner. This naturally confused his results. He went on to say, in support of his prophecy, that "life is speedily destroyed by from 20 to 25 per cent."

As I have personally given ethylene in about 1,100 cases, very often at a concentration of about 88 per cent., without ill-effects, I am quite sure that these other factors were very important in misleading Mr. Nunneley.

He also claimed that

"coal gas is not only a powerful anæsthetic, but, so far as my experiments go, it is also a very safe and manageable one." " . . . when other agents are not to hand . . . no hesitation need be felt in employing this substance."

Here the key lies in the words "so far as my experiments go," for this somewhat risky advice was given on the strength of six experiments only. He went on . . . "if in practice it should be found, as I believe it will, to be successful, the cheapness of the method would be a recommendation." This dangerous insistence on cheapness was still in operation a hundred years later, unfortunately.

Other predictions made by Mr. Nunneley were very far from the truth.

"Ether, which . . . was for some time almost exclusively used, has now almost ceased to be employed . . . it will hereafter, I apprehend, be rarely used." Protoxide of nitrogen (N_2O) " . . . appeared to well deserve a trial."

But his experiments, five of them only, were

"quite sufficient to show that nitrous oxide never could be employed as an anæsthetic, and that the inhalation of it is not altogether so harmless as is generally supposed."

Again, his tests of this gas were carried out by putting small animals in jars of it. As oxygen was not present the time factor in taking them out was very important.

W. de C. Wheeler,[10] referring to Crile's anociassociation method of preventing shock, made the rash prophecy that general anæsthesia would disappear altogether, in other than exceptional cases. These inaccurate forecasts are not confined to any one era or decade. They occur throughout the whole history of anæsthesia. Nicholas Ivanovitch Pirogoff, in the very early days, when he introduced rectal ether in 1847, said: "It seems to me that this method will completely replace the pneumatic method."[11]

All the above examples illustrate the extreme uncertainty of any attempt to foretell the future. Potential prophets should always remember that a very numerous and prosperous tribe of bookmakers and turf accountants have for many years made their living out of this simple fact.

References

[1] Sir John Eric Erichson (1873). *Lancet,* Oct. 4.
[2] Sir St. Clair Thomson (1938). *Lancet,* Oct. 15. 911.
[3] M. Velpeau (1839). *Médicine Opératoire.* Vol. 1, p. 32. Paris.
[4] M. Velpeau (1847). *Comptes Rendus Lbd. Acad. Sci.* Paris. 76.
[5] C. T. Jackson (1861). *A Manual of Etherization.* Boston: Mansfield.
[6] Ranyard West (1935). *Proc. R. Soc. Med.* 28. 565.
[7] G. P. Pitkin (1929). *Brit. med. J.,* Aug. 3. 183.
[8] Thomas Jonnesco (1909). *Brit. med. J.,* Nov. 13. 1401.
[9] Thomas Nunneley (1849). *Trans. Prov. med. surg. Ass.* Vol. XVI. 167.
[10] W. de C. Wheeler (1914). *Brit. med. J.,* Aug. 22. 354.
[11] *Comptes Rendus Lbd. Acad. Sci.* Paris. (1847), 5th May seance. 789.

CHAPTER 14

THE DEATH OF MISS IDA WYNDHAM, NITROUS OXIDE'S FIRST VICTIM

Lancet, 1873, Feb. 1. 178. Death from nitrous oxide.

At Exeter on Jan. 22nd, Mr. J. T. Browne Mason, dentist, gave gas to Miss Ida Wyndham, aged 38, for extraction of an upper molar. The pulse became rapid, and Dr. Pattison, who was present, thought less full, while she was still conscious. The inhaler was taken away and an attempt at extraction made, but she could not bear it. Gas was given again. Her face became swollen and livid. She died. No post-mortem.

A fortnight later there was a letter from F. Woodhouse Braine, who was born in 1837 and qualified in 1858. When Henry Potter retired Braine became the only other pure anæsthetist besides Clover. He was twenty-one years at the Dental Hospital, and among the first to use nitrous oxide in this country. He was the first anæsthetist at Charing Cross Hospital and worked there for eighteen years. He used the Ormsby inhaler for ether. He died on October 28th, 1907, in his seventy-first year. His son, Charles Carter Braine, also became anæsthetist to Charing Cross Hospital. This letter was written about five years after T. W. Evans's first demonstration of gas anæsthesia in this country.

Lancet, 1873, Feb. 15. 253.

After saying that the newspaper reports were unreliable Braine said that he did not believe that the patient died from the effects of the gas. "What Dr. Pattison really does say is, and I quote from the report drawn up by him in conjunction with Dr. Drake and Mr. Browne Mason, 'that the pulse became less rapid, but that its volume did not vary'." The *Lancet* had said that death was clearly due to paralysis of the respiration, and that there was no obstruction to the air passages. "This is not true, for there was considerable enlargement of both tonsils, with chronic elongation of the uvula interfering with her breathing, and rendering it at times somewhat loud." There was no entry of air into the chest on artificial respiration. Had there been paralysis of respiration, this would not have prevented the entry of air.

Lancet, 1873, Feb. 15. 254.

Abstract of report by Mr. Browne Mason. The patient was stout, with enlarged tonsils, prominent eyes and an underhung jaw. Her breathing was loud and snorting on exertion (? exophthalmic goitre). The bleeding after the first attempt was very slight. There was no cyanosis on removing the inhaler for the second time. There was a ten minute interval since the first attempt. All fragments were accounted for, and none of them went down the throat. The wooden gag was difficult to remove and was found later to be chipped. It was not known whether it was chipped before the anæsthesia. No blood went down the throat. The heart beat for two minutes after the respiration had ceased. The sounds produced during artificial respiration were only those of expiration. Dr. Pattison was Miss Wyndham's brother-in-law. There was no P.M.

There follows, ten months later, an interesting letter from G. Q. Colton, who was by far the most prominent figure in the world of nitrous oxide in the pre-McKesson era.

Lancet, 1873, Dec. 13. 857. Letter from G. Q. Colton, New York.

Sir,—In the February number of your valuable journal, an article appears under the heading of "A case of fatal suffocation from nitrous oxide gas," which in my opinion contains so many errors regarding the operation and effects of the gas that I ask space for this reply.

In regard to the death of Miss Wyndham, which you so circumstantially describe, the question is whether she died from the effects of the gas, or from the unfortunate treatment she received after having fainted, and after the effects of the gas had passed off. You state: "She took the gas in the usual way, without any symptoms to excite uneasiness. At the proper degree of insensibility the inhalation was stopped, and the tooth was extracted. In the operation Mr. Mason was obliged to split the fangs and take them out separately. It was not until after the operation was completed that anything unusual happened, but immediately afterwards the face became livid. . . . Mr. Mason hastened to fetch Dr. Drake, who returned with him, and who found the lady still alive. She was sitting in a chair in a half-reclined position, before an open window.

It will be observed that she fainted "after the operation was completed." She certainly could not have fainted while under the influence of the gas, because, from the extra supply of oxygen in the gas, the action of the heart and the circulation of the blood is increased rather than arrested. Indeed the gas is the quickest and surest remedy to administer in cases of fainting. If this lady had been placed at once flat upon the floor, and some water dashed in her face, in all probability she would have revived. There are many cases on record where patients have died in the dentist's chair when no anæsthetic was administered. Why assume that this death was caused by the gas, when nothing unusual happened till after the effects of the gas had passed off?

The great mistake of the *Lancet* is contained in the following extracts:— "From no agent have there been so many hairbreadth escapes from death as from this gas, and probably of late some persons every day have been brought within the minutest line of the danger to which Miss Wyndham succumbed. . . . Nitrous oxide, indeed, is not an anæsthetic at all. A true anæsthetic is an agent which suspends common sensibility without, by any necessity, interfering with those organic processes on the continuance of which life depends. Nitrous oxide acts, not in this way, but by suspending for a brief period one of the most important of the organic processes—that of respiration itself."

In reply to the first extract, I have to say that it is a mere assertion without any proof. The *Lancet* admits that this is the *only* death which has occurred in England from the effects of the gas, and I think I have shown that even this case cannot with certainty be attributed to the gas. The gas has been administered many years and by hundreds of dentists in England. How can it, then, be assumed that "some persons every day have been brought within the minutest line" of death? Practical experience is better than theory in such a matter.

In regard to the second extract, in which it is stated that nitrous oxide is not an anæsthetic, and that it suspends respiration, I have to answer, the *Lancet never made a greater mistake.* I speak from an experience of over ten years in administering the gas, and to over 67,000 patients. I have given the gas for something over a hundred operations in general surgery, in which I have kept patients in the anæsthetic sleep from five to sixteen consecutive minutes; and have the testimony of the distinguished surgeon, Dr. J. Marion Sims, that he has performed operations with the gas where the insensibility was continued over one hour.. According to the reasoning of the *Lancet,* respiration (breathing) was suspended during all this time! No one can question the fact that the gas will produce insensibility to pain.

And now as to the safety of the gas as an anæsthetic. I presume it is known that I introduced the gas (or rather revived it) to the dental profession in July, 1863. After using it for about nine months, I commenced to ask my patients to write their names on a scroll. These names I have numbered regularly from the beginning. The number on the scroll at this writing is *sixty-seven thousand, four hundred and fifty-five* (67,455).

It should be added that Colton, by 1881, during a period of seventeen years, had raised his scroll numbers to the astonishing total of 121,709 without a death.[1]

In all this vast number I have never had a fatal case, or even a case of serious injury, from the effects of the gas. We have an occasional case of vomiting—not oftener than one in a hundred—and this, usually, from swallowing a little blood. During the past eight years we have averaged from twenty to thirty patients every day, and occasionally reaching fifty. In the spring of 1868 I exhibited to a large number of leading dentists and surgeons in London, at the office of Mr. Charles James Fox, the autograph signatures of *over nineteen thousand of the above patients.*

What do these facts prove? Not that "the administration of nitrous oxide is a harmless process—a process which any man, educated or uneducated, may carry out without danger of destroying life." No one pretends this. But it shows that, with ordinary care and prudence, it is a comparatively safe agent, even in the hands of ordinary dentists. There are many thousands of dentists in the United States who have used the gas during the past eight or nine years, so that it is safe to assume that three hundred thousand have inhaled it in this country for teeth extraction, and yet *not a death has occurred!* (There was a *reported* death from the effects of the gas in this city, but on investigation it was shown that the patient only *attempted* to breathe the gas three or four times, and finally concluded to have her eight teeth drawn without it, which was done. She fainted from the pain and shock, and unfortunately, like Miss Wyndham, was kept in an upright position for some ten minutes. In referring to this case, the *Lancet* admitted the "ineffectual" attempts to administer the gas, and stated that the patient would probably have recovered if she had been laid flat on the floor. In my opinion, if this woman had inhaled the gas properly she would have been alive today.)

To use any anæsthetic successfully requires experience. It does not of necessity require great knowledge in chemistry or surgery. If any of your learned readers were to stand by my chair and see me administer the gas successfully to a hundred patients, though I profess no great scientific knowledge, he would prefer to trust himself in my hands in a similar operation upon himself, rather than rely upon the theoretical knowledge of any physician or surgeon, however distinguished.

The difference in the action of nitrous oxide and chloroform is, that chloroform, containing no oxygen, arrests or retards the action of the heart, and really carries the patient *towards* the point of death; and about one in 2,500 die from it. Nitrous oxide, containing more oxygen than the atmospheric air, increases the action of the heart, and carries the patient into increased and higher life. One gives life, the other death. At least half a million people (the world over) have taken the gas for teeth extracting and not a death has occurred, or only one, according to the *Lancet*. It appears to me that if experiments are to be made with a view to "learn" how to use anæsthetics, they should be made with that agent which has been proved to be the most safe. In view of all the above facts, no one can question that nitrous oxide, in point of safety, is vastly superior to all known anæsthetics. Dentists who commence the use of the gas often make the mistake of not administering enough, or of having too small a passage for the patient to breathe through; but these are errors which time and experience will correct. I am, Sir, your obedient servant, G. Q. Colton. New York, Aug. 18th, 1873.

P.S.—The *Lancet* states that the pulse of the patient became rapid under the influence of the gas, as though this was an unfavourable symptom. The rapidity of the pulse (in health) depends upon the rapidity with which it is oxygenised in the lungs. When we run upstairs, or engage in any sudden muscular exertion, we breathe faster, and supply oxygen to the lungs faster, thus preparing it more rapidly for circulation. There is a corresponding increase in the rapidity of the pulse. The nitrous oxide, being composed of one half oxygen, supplies this oxygen to the lungs so rapidly that the pulse is increased by fifteen or twenty beats in a minute when it is given for anæsthesia. If the operation is attended with great mental excitement, the pulse may be increased thirty or forty beats, not certainly reaching a point of danger.

A person *can* "hold the breath" for a considerable time after inhaling the gas, because an extra quantity of oxygen is suddenly supplied to the lungs. The blood continues to flow till the extra oxygen is used up. The pearl-divers take a dozen or twenty rapid and deep inhalations of common air and then go under water and remain a long time, until the extra oxygen supplied to the lungs is exhausted. By this rapid and deep inhalation of common air a person can make the head swim, or put himself into a half anæsthetic condition. The gas does the same thing, only carrying the effect a little further.

Comment by the Lancet:

Our correspondent, by the very candour which he exhibits, prevents us from replying to him as we might have been tempted to reply. He takes credit only for what he calls practical knowledge, and professes "no great scientific knowledge". This is to be regretted, because he offers observations purporting to be scientific—that is to say, to be based on scientific fact or observation. We, on our part, have a practical knowledge of anæsthesia as extended as it can be, insomuch as it extends from the first days of the introduction of the art to the present day without a break in our labour of any serious duration. But we have striven also to get at principles; we have experimented to learn; and we thereupon came to a difference with Dr. Colton on vital points. We assert, on facts gained both by experience and experiment, that the lady who died at Exeter from nitrous oxide did not die of syncope, that she showed no sign of syncope, but that she died of asphyxia. We assert, on like evidence, that nitrous oxide is not decomposed in the human body, and that there is no proof whatever that the oxygen it contains is applied for oxidation in the organism. We suggest, on good evidence, that the rapid pulse which follows the administration of the gas is due not to stimulation of the heart, but to the resistance which is taken off the heart from an induced paralysis of the vessels of the minute circulation; and we affirm that a man or an animal can live longer with the lungs filled with common air than with the same organs filled with nitrous oxide. In a word, Dr. Colton's experiences of administration, which we do not dispute, show that asphyxia can be carried to the point of inducing insensibility with fewer accidents than might be supposed. The experiments in the Grotto del Cane prove the same fact; and we remember that, some years ago, when, on an enquiry into the management of one of our great English institutions for the insane, it was shown that for years upon years certain troublesome patients had been systematically quieted, before their washing and dressing, by the process of compressing their wind-pipes by a few twists of a soft stocking, it was contended that the process never did any harm. These facts, in their bearing on asphyxia, are most valuable, as are also some others which illustrate that a living body may be submerged in water several minutes, and may yet recover after removal; but they have nothing directly to do with anæsthesia, as a scientific study. Perfect anæsthesia is, in principle, the art of suspending sensations and sensibility, without interfering with those processes upon which the continuance of life depends. The administration of a gas which stops the process of respiration, though it suspends sensation and sensibility for a short period prior to death, is no part of this perfected art; and we shall persist, notwithstanding Dr. Colton's practical knowledge, in upholding the principle of scientific investigation until the art is perfected.—Ed., *L.*

Colton—not Dr. Colton, for he was never medically qualified—is of course quite wrong about the oxygen content of nitrous oxide. He assumes it to be free oxygen, available to the body, as in ordinary air. The *Lancet* corrects this erroneous view.

We shall see later how Courville based a perfectly correct principle on completely invalid and irrelevant evidence. We now have the position reversed. Colton, a most experienced and successful user of nitrous oxide, who had, at this time, an experience of 67,455 cases (which he increased to 121,709 by 1881[1]) without a single death, based his correct practice on an entirely erroneous principle.

It is not altogether surprising that he could do this in the short dental 'fill-ups' which composed the vast majority of his cases. Such is the inherent safety and non-toxicity of the gas that the average patient can be taken almost to the point of respiratory arrest—and will recover directly air is given. But Colton went beyond this in a few cases. So great was his empirical skill that he even gave long gas anæsthesias—up to sixteen minutes, according to his own statement—for surgical operations. Nothing is said about the addition of oxygen, so these administrations must have been intermittent, with frequent breaths of air allowed.

This being so, it is singular that he did not discover his mistake about the available oxygen content of nitrous oxide, for in these long cases—about 100 of them—he must have found that pure gas could not be given continuously, but that air had to be given at intervals; and that air had an oxygenating effect infinitely greater than that supposedly due to nitrous oxide, which was, in fact, nil.

The *Lancet* correctly points out this mistake, but falls into error itself in referring to nitrous oxide as a gas which stops the process of respiration. The gas can be correctly described as an oxygen replacing agent, which interferes with oxygen metabolism, but to say that it arrested respiration was mere foolishness in view of Colton's immense series of cases which were unique in anæsthesia for the very reason that, alone among anæsthetics, respiratory arrest had never occurred. In fact the total condemnation of gas by the *Lancet* goes too far, and is much too sweeping.

The death of Miss Wyndham seems to have been due to asphyxia, as far as one can judge, not from the gas alone, but from the gas combined with many unfavourable circumstances. Her face was livid and swollen. She had enlarged tonsils and an enlarged uvula. She was stout, with an underhung jaw, and quite possibly an enlarged thyroid with pressure on the trachea—she is described as having prominent eyes and snorting or noisy breathing on exertion. There had been some bleeding from the first abortive attempt at extraction—it was stated to be slight, but it might have been more profuse than was thought, taking into account the ten minutes which elapsed between the two attempts and the fact that some of the blood might have disappeared into the air-passages. Added to all this she probably had tight corsets on. All these little things add up; besides the missing fragment of gag might have been impacted in the larynx. Nobody looked to see.

Reference

[1] Henry M. Lyman (1882). *Artificial Anæsthesia and Anæsthetics.*

CHAPTER 15

AN INTESTINAL INTERLUDE

NICHOLAS IVANOVITCH PIROGOFF (1810-1881), of St. Petersburg (later Petrograd, now Leningrad), had an original idea in the early days of ether. Instead of using it by inhalation in the ordinary way he turned to the other end of the patient and administered it per rectum. This he did for the first time on April 2nd, 1847,[1] less than six months after Ether Day. He has always had an unchallenged priority in this respect.

Then I found a reference which raised doubts in my mind.[2] Dr. J. T. Johnstone used ether vapour by the same route in Madras at about the same time. A copy of the *Madras Spectator* reported the case, and the *Lancet* quoted it from that source. It was a case of hydrocele. One ounce of ether was placed in a bladder fitted with an ivory pipe. The bladder was dipped in hot water and the vapour injected into the rectum. The patient stated that it felt "like an injection of boiling lead" and refused to go on with it. He had the operation without anæsthesia, so he must have felt very strongly about the matter. The only other point mentioned is that he passed many dead worms during the next week. The exact date is not given, so it has to be deduced as nearly as possible from the facts which we do know. The report appeared in the *Lancet* of July 10th, so the question at once arises, what was the shortest possible time for the news to travel from India to England?

The Records department of the General Post Office gave me some useful information here.

> "Under ordinary circumstances the length of voyages at that time were from Calcutta 48 days, from Madras 45 days. The mails were scheduled for despatch from Sandheads, Calcutta, on the 10th day of the month and from Madras on the 12th day of the month, arriving at Southampton on 26th day of the month. The arrival date of mail from India to England before 10th July would therefore be 26th June, and this would necessitate despatching from India on 10th or 12th May."

Hence the Indian operation must have dated from a day or two before the 12th May. Presumably not long before, or the item would have lost its news value for the local press. Suppose we say 10th May, which is as near as we are likely to get. This still leaves Pirogoff with his priority by a margin of thirty-eight days.

The next point to investigate is, could Dr. Johnstone have heard the news from St. Petersburg in the time, or was he an entirely independent pioneer of the method? The Post Office letter continues:

"in the absence of any information relating to the transit times of mail from Russia to India we are unable to express any opinion as to the time taken for news of the demonstration on 2nd April, 1847, by Ivanovitch Pirogoff to reach India. . . ."

If the Post Office don't know it is going to be difficult, if not impossible, to reach any certainty in this matter. It is a fair assumption, however, that if the mails took 45 days from Madras to England, they would take considerably longer from St. Petersburg to Madras. The sea voyage is a good deal longer, and it is very unlikely that there was any rapid north to south overland transport in Russia at that time—not to mention the problem of crossing the mighty barrier of the Himalayan mountains. If this reasoning is correct then Dr. Johnstone must have had the idea *de novo*. He could not possibly have heard about Pirogoff's work in the thirty-eight days available.

As a last hope of getting further information about postal services in Russia in the 1840s I wrote to the Soviet Union Embassy in London. I know the Russians are not very good at answering questions, particularly vital ones which affect the lives of all inhabitants of this planet, but it is just possible that on a point of this nature, which is of no practical importance to anybody, but which admits Russian priority in one tiny corner of science, they may really spread themselves. I half expect to receive a copy of Pirogoff's book and perhaps a free trip to Petrograd! We shall see.

I got a reply in eight days. The Ambassador passed my letter on to their Press Service, and Mr. Donovan Brown answered it very fully and very courteously.

"I see your point, but I am afraid we cannot be of great assistance. The first railway open in Russia was a very short line between Petersburg and Tsarskoye in 1837, but I have no reference available which would give me the dates for longer lines giving possible contact with India. The Trans-Siberian line did not come into being until a year or two before the Russo-Japanese War of 1904."

(According to Nelson's Dictionary of Dates it was begun in 1891, and the Manchurian section, or E. Chinese Railway, completed in 1901.)

"Neither have I references giving any indication of the transport of mails from Russia to India in 1847. What is now the Asiatic Republics was, in those days, so undeveloped and transport so rudimentary, that I cannot think a letter would travel through India, Afghanistan, through what are largely desert regions in Russia, and on to the North. An alternative route across the Arabian Sea, Persian Gulf, Iraq, Turkey, the Caucasus would be no quicker, and the most likely route appears to be the longest—round the Cape and up the Baltic, probably to Riga, for in those days, as again, the Baltic provinces were part of Russia. Riga is free of ice a month before Leningrad (St. Petersburg) so it might depend on what time a ship arrived, whether it put post ashore at Riga, or went straight to St. Petersburg. I am sorry we cannot be more helpful on this occasion. We could, of course, make research in Moscow, but I am afraid this would take rather a long time and I do not know how pressing is your enquiry."

On the whole the information, though rather vague, is as detailed as one can expect. It was a small and unimportant incident, and it happened a long time ago, so I doubt if Moscow would be able to give any more definite answers. Such as they are the details tend to support the conclusion I had previously arrived at, that the news could not possibly have got through from North Russia to India in thirty-eight days, by any route, at that time. This makes Dr. Johnstone an independent discoverer of the method, and also leaves Pirogoff as the pioneer by a small margin.

Then I found another reference, in an article by W. T. G. Morton himself.[3] On turning, by his advice, to *Comptes Rendus hebdomadaires de l'Academie des Sciences* for 1847 I found that at least one other person had been working on the same method, at about the same time. M. Marc-Dupuy used the rectal method experimentally early enough to have his results published at the meeting on the 5th April,[4] one month before Pirogoff's first article on the subject, which was read at the next meeting on 5th May. So Marc-Dupuy appears to have priority of publication at least, though he does not mention the use of the method in human beings. Pirogoff also states that he first tried it out on animals. Later, in time for the June meeting Pirogoff's book arrived, with a letter detailing further cases.

Note on the effects of the injection of ether into the rectum, by M. Marc-Dupuy. Translated by the author. (W.S.S.)[4]

"I wished to find out if it was not possible to introduce ether into the economy by another route than the lungs, in order to avoid the disadvantages attached to this method. The experience I have had with three dogs and a rabbit have demonstrated that ether injected into the rectum is absorbed with great rapidity, and that it results in complete insensibility. The alteration in colour of the arterial blood, which one notices in inhalation etherisation and which denotes that asphyxia is more or less advanced, does not take place when ether is injected into the rectum."

Experiment with a dog.

"I injected into the rectum of a small sized dog a mixture of 15 grammes of sulphuric ether and 15 grammes of water, after having briskly shaken the two liquids together. The animal had not eaten for seven or eight hours. At the end of one minute the breath had a very pronounced smell of ether; there came from the mouth some frothy saliva, in a fair quantity. Four minutes after the injection drunkenness was complete; the animal could not remain on its feet; it was only by dragging itself on the ground that it could change its position. Insensibility was complete; I made sure of this by transfixing the skin with pins; an incision made in the skin with a bistoury caused no pain.

"Eleven minutes elapsed, the drunkenness persisted: the animal in the meantime began to be able to hold itself upright, but when it wished to walk it fell at every step. Very complete insensibility still existed; at the end of eighteen minutes walking was easier but the drunkenness had not yet wholly passed off. Sensibility began to return, for, on piercing the skin with pins there was a slight contraction of the paucier."

I could not find this last word in any of the dozen French dictionaries which I consulted, so I cannot tell you what contracted. Even the large *Littré* does not give it.

"Although meanwhile the animal had not made any complaints it seemed to be completely unconcerned about what one did.

"At the end of twenty-two minutes, sensibility had reappeared; the animal walked with assurance, the inebriation did not exist any more; only then did it vomit a small quantity of a frothy liquid with no special characteristics.

"During the whole time the experiment lasted, nothing was passed *per anum*. There was a fairly abundant salivation. The animal snapped continually. As the drunkenness had passed off I gave him some food, and he ate with a good appetite. This injection of ether and water only caused slight irritation of the mucosa of the large intestine, for the animal had only a little diarrhoea."

Experiment with a rabbit.

"I injected into the rectum of a rabbit a mixture of 10 grammes of ether and 10 grammes of water. At the end of three minutes insensibility was complete. I then wished to examine the blood; I cut the two femoral arteries one by one, immediately there came out perfectly normal red blood. I then opened the abdomen, making an incision starting at the base of the chest and going as far as the symphysis pubis; the animal, at the moment when I completed the incision, made a slight movement, which made me think that the inebriation was beginning to pass off; I at once gave another injection of ether and water, and from then the most perfect insensibility persisted during the whole period of the experiment. I took out the intestines from the abdominal cavity and soon got to the aorta, which I cut across. The blood was a ruddy red and came out in spurts. I opened the chest: the heart was still beating, but feebly; the lungs were pink and did not show the least trace of engorgement; the spleen, the liver and the kidneys did not show anything abnormal; the intestines contained very little gas; there was not the least trace of injection of the rectal mucosa.

"This observation proves, I think, in a most satisfactory way, that insensibility is by no means the necessary result of asphyxia, as some experimenters have asserted. . . ."

The French here becomes obscure and beyond my powers of translation, so a chunk of it is omitted.

"I do not deny that asphyxia would be an excellent means of destroying sensibility, but I doubt that anybody would be tempted to employ it a first time, for fear of not being able to do it again.

"To sum up, I believe it to be true to say:

"1. That sensibility is abolished when one injects ether into the rectum.

"2. That the etherisation takes place as quickly as when one introduces ether into the economy by the lungs.

"3. That there are no signs of asphyxia.

"4. That this method can be employed with greater safety than that which consists in causing the vapour of ether to be respired."

"Nouveau procédé pour produire, au moyen de la vapeur d'éther, l'insensibilité chez les individus soumis à des operations chirurgicales."

Extract from a letter from M. Pirogoff, Professor of Clinical Surgery at the Imperial Academy at St. Petersburg.[5] Translated by the author (W.S.S.).

"This method consists in the introduction of the vapour of ether by the rectum. The experiments I have made on animals have authorised me to use it in surgical operations, even in cases where inhalation of ether has been used on the patient without the least success."

Here, as in the case of Velpeau, we can trace the beginnings of the continental attitude to anæsthesia. If the thing doesn't work perfectly the first time, don't bother to learn how to do it. There isn't anything to learn. Try something else.

"After clearing the lower part of the intestinal canal by a simple wash-out, I insert a flexible tube (une sonde élastique) into the rectum, and I fit to the end of this tube, by means of a screw, the syringe which I also use for blood transfusion. The syringe is contained in a 'capsule' of tin, which is filled with water at 40° Reaumur (122° F., 50° C.). Thanks to this arrangement, the liquid ether, which is introduced from the bottle into the syringe, passes at once from the liquid state to the state of vapour, and it is in this form that it enters, by the flexible tube, into the rectum."

Pirogoff does not appear to have had the trouble experienced by Dr. Johnstone in India, whose patient stated that the vapour injection was so painful that he preferred to dispense with anæsthesia altogether and have the operation done without.

"The advantages of this method are evident; the organs of respiration do not suffer at all. The etherisation is completely independent of the will of the patient, and it acts much more promptly; after two to four minutes the respired air already smells very strongly of ether. It seems to me that this method will completely replace the pneumatic method (which is) very often inconvenient and painful to the patients. Operations whose performance with the pneumatic method has been very difficult, as, for example, many operations on the face, on the mouth, and above all, operations in infants, can now be accomplished very easily by my method.

"The quantity of ether, in the cases observed by me, up to the present, was only 1½ to 2 ounces, and the narcotisation was ordinarily complete after three to five minutes. Up to the present, there have never been any unpleasant results."

As Pirogoff does not say whether he has used the method in 6 cases or 6,000, his last sentence is not really very helpful.

Abstract of letter from Pirogoff, who sent it, and a copy of his book, to the meeting of 21st June.[6]

Since the publication of his book he had had the opportunity of applying his method with complete success in some more cases. Twice for partial removal of the upper jaw—the patients were perfectly drowsy but very easily got rid of the blood and mucus which collected in the mouth and throat during the operation. Five times for eye operations, which were made easier by the immobility of the eye. In one of the cases the eye turned upwards but was hooked by the conjunctiva and drawn down. One case of rhinoplasty lasted three quarters of an hour, and the anæsthesia lasted out long enough. Once for removal of metacarpals and once for cutting for the stone.

In all the cases the feverish and nervous reaction after the operation was no worse than usual, and the drowsiness came on without excitement. In one case excitement came on during recovery.

These early articles are interesting, but the problem of who was really the first to think of the idea is, to me, insoluble. All we can say is that M. Marc-Dupuy, Pirogoff and Dr. J. T. Johnstone were practically neck and neck.

References

[1] N. I. Pirogoff (1847). *Recherches pratiques et physiologiques sur l'etherisation.* St. Petersburg.
[2] *Lancet* (1847), July 10. 50.
[3] W. T. G. Morton (1850). *Boston med. surg. J.* Vol. 43. 109.
[4] *C. R. Acad. Sci. Paris* (1847), 5th April seance. 605.
[5] (1847), 5th May seance. 789.
[6] (1847), 21st June seance. 1110.

CHAPTER 16

CHLOROFORM BEFORE SIMPSON;

An Indian Medical Service Claimant

Soon after the death of Sir James Simpson, which took place on 6th May, 1870, a letter appeared in the *Lancet*[1] from Michael Cudmore Furnell, F.R.C.S., Surgeon, H.M.'s Indian Army, Professor of Physiology, Madras Medical College. It was dated February, 1871. The letter is quoted in full elsewhere.[2] It is a short letter, but makes the claim that the writer used chloroform before it was introduced to the profession by Simpson. Seven years later the same man wrote to the *Lancet* again, a long article this time, giving a more complete account of this interesting and important challenge. The great detail of the story and the evidence quoted in it makes it very certain that it was genuine.[3]

Some remarks on the discovery of the anæsthetic effects of chloroform, and its first exhibition in England. M. C. Furnell, M.D., F.R.C.S., Surgeon-major, H.M.'s Indian Service, Principal of the Madras Medical College, etc.

"I have no desire whatever in the following remarks to attempt to snatch a single laurel from the wreath of fame which enriches the brow of Sir James Simpson. To his other merits, as one of the most able and famous medical men of his time, Sir James Simpson has had added the reputation of having first discovered, and then introduced to the world, the use of chloroform as an anæsthetic. That he first introduced it in Edinburgh, and by his example, and owing to his eminent position, made the use of chloroform quickly and widely popular throughout the civilised world, is a matter which admits of, and happily needs, no denial, but I think I shall be able to show in the following remarks that five or six months before Sir James Simpson used this beneficent agent, it had been first taken, and then brought to the notice of two eminent hospital surgeons of London by the writer of these lines, then a young student just commencing the study of medicine.

"The subject has not only been noticed by Dr. Edward S. Dunster in his paper 'The History of Anæsthesia,' but has lately formed a topic of discussion in one of the leading daily papers of the presidency in which I am serving, and the statements there made by a correspondent signing himself 'X.Y.Z.' led me to make some inquiries in the matter full of interest to myself, and not without interest, I hope, to the medical profession.

"I will first relate, as concisely as I can, my connexion with this discovery of the anæsthetic properties of chloroform, how it lay buried so many years, and how the subject was again resuscitated.

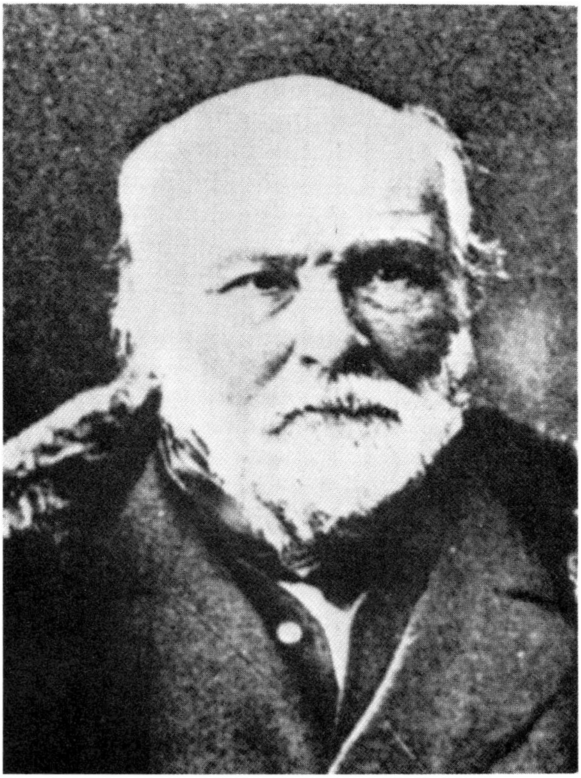

PLATE XLVI

Nikolai Ivanovitch Pirogoff. 1810-1881. Born November 13 at Moscow. Qualified 1833 at Dorpat. 1836-1840 Professor of Surgery at Dorpat. 1840 Professor of Clinical Surgery, St. Petersburg. At Sevastopol during the Crimean War, had to give up his professorship because of his criticisms of the War Department. Usually credited with being the first to use rectal ether, but M. Marc-Dupuy and J. T. Johnstone used the method at about the same time.

From *Introduction to the History of Medicine*. Fielding H. Garrison. 1913. Philadelphia: W. B. Saunders Co.

"It was in the year 1846 that Dr. Morton of Boston made known his grand discovery of anæsthesia by sulphuric ether, one of the most astounding revolutions in medicine. Before this time, to use the words of Velpeau, 'a cutting instrument and pain in operative surgery were inseparably connected in the minds of patients, and there seemed no appeal from this apparent necessary association'. Men who can remember the operation theatre of a large hospital before Dr. Morton's discovery are gradually passing away; they are every day becoming fewer. (Written 31 years after the discovery.) I can well remember even now one of the first operations I saw under the old *régime*. It was on a girl who had in childhood been desperately burnt on the neck and shoulders by falling into a fire. The cicatrix had gradually contracted, so as to draw the unfortunate creature's head down on her breast and her lower lip away from the mouth, exposing the lower row of teeth and allowing the saliva to dribble continually from her mouth. She was a repulsive spectacle, and had gladly consented to Mr. Skey's suggestion of an operation, which by transplanting a piece of skin from her arm and dissecting up the cicatrix, appeared to afford some chance of mitigating her unfortunate appearance. The patient was tied to the operating table, as was customary in those days, but before many minutes of the operation had elapsed, her cries and entreaties to be untied and allowed to remain as she was were the most frightful that can be imagined. As the operation, which was necessarily a lengthy and slow one, proceeded, her cries became more terrible; first one and then another student fainted, and ultimately all but a determined few had left the theatre unable to stand the distressing scene. I have since that time assisted, as the French say, at some painful sights. I have seen a strong man flogged for gross insubordination in the field, but his sufferings were light as air compared with the agonies this poor girl must have undergone. These terrible scenes in the operating theatre of a hospital were of weekly, almost daily occurrence, when Dr. Morton's merciful discovery, like the wand of a beneficent fairy, swept them for ever from the world. Has the enormous and priceless benefit of his discovery ever been rightly appreciated by mankind? I am afraid not.

"It was in the year 1846 that I commenced my studies for a surgeon. I had not been intended for the profession of medicine, so that I discovered, shortly after I began, that not having been pupiled or apprenticed to a practitioner, as was customary in those days, would be a bar to my presenting myself for examination at the College of Surgeons. To overcome this it was necessary to produce a certificate of having attended a course of practical pharmacy, and for this purpose I became a pupil of Mr. Jacob Bell. It was whilst attending his laboratory that the medical world became agitated with the startling discovery of Dr. Morton, and numberless instruments were devised and manufactured for the safe or more effectual administration of sulphuric ether. I, with the inquisitiveness of a youth of seventeen, enthusiastic in his profession, used to amuse myself trying these new instruments and passing my verdict upon them. At last Mr. Bell, alarmed no doubt at the possibility of some accident occurring, gave orders that I was not to be allowed this indiscriminate use of ether, and I found my experiments suddenly cut short. It was on the occurrence of this failure of sulphuric ether that one day, looking about for some to try on a new instrument, I came across a bottle labelled chloric ether. It was a covered and neglected bottle, away in a dark storeroom. Its contents smelt pleasant, and I, with the audacity of seventeen, put some into the instrument and commenced its inhalation. I soon discovered that it was a much more pleasant substance than sulphuric ether. It had a sweetish, agreeable taste, and did not cause that irritative, suffocative cough which made the inhalation of sulphuric ether so unpleasant and to some patients impossible. It soon also began to produce insensibility.

"I drew Mr. Bell's attention to this new discovery, and he recommended me to take it down to St. Bartholomew's Hospital and bring it to the notice of the surgeons there. What followed is best told, perhaps, in Mr. Holmes Coote's own words, as quoted by Sir R. Christison:—'In the summer of 1847 Sir William Lawrence operated on a lady in Essex for scirrhus of the breast, and I accompanied him to assist him and to give the patient sulphuric ether. She coughed so violently that I had great difficulty in obtaining the necessary anæsthetic effects. Some week or so afterwards I was talking about the inconvenience in the hospital (St. Bartholomew's), when a Mr. Furnell, now in the Bengal Army,* told me he had a milder anæsthetic, commonly called chloric ether, which he advised me to try. With Sir William Lawrence's assent I used it several times in private practice, and once upon the lady who had such trouble with sulphuric ether, and we invariably found that the effect, though slow, was free from other inconveniences.' My own recollection of the matter is that I took the bottle down and showed it to Mr. Holmes Coote. He was at that time demonstrator of anatomy, and a great favourite with us all from his kindly and genial manner—just the man a young student would have gone to to communicate such a matter. He asked me if I could guarantee its safety, and my reply was that I had taken it myself, and was none the worse. This was in 1847. My own impression is that it was in the month of May; I am not, however, at this distance of time, quite sure of the month, but it was in the spring time.

"In due course of time I passed the College, and went out to India in the medical service of the old Honourable East India Company. The fact that I had used and introduced this chloric ether to the notice of Mr. Holmes Coote and Sir William Lawrence I had in no way forgotten, and often mentioned in conversation with medical friends, but no more notice of the matter seemed to me at all necessary.

"In 1869 I came home to England on furlough, and the following strange *rencontre* took place. I, one Sunday, went down to All Saints, Margaret Street,

*This was a mistake of Mr. Holmes Coote; he should have written Madras Army.

the famous ritualistic church, to escort home a lady, a relative of mine. There, bound, I subsequently discovered, on a similar errand, I saw Mr. Holmes Coote. I had not seen him certainly for sixteen or seventeen years, but his was a face not easily forgotten. I addressed him: 'How do you do, Mr. Coote? You have no doubt forgotten me, but I remember you very well. I am an old Bartholomew's man'. He looked at me for a moment, and then said, 'I remember you; your name is Nell—nell something; you are the man who gave me the chloroform many years ago; do you remember?' 'Oh, yes, I remember very well, chloric ether; my name is Furnell.' 'Ah! Furnell, that's it; do you remember? Confound it, what simpletons we were not to have proclaimed our discovery. Why, we had chloroform some months before Sir James Simpson'. I laughed at his enthusiasm, and subsequently went home to his house, and had luncheon, and a pleasant chat over old times.

"It was whilst I was at home on this furlough that Sir James Simpson died, and I subsequently sent a short note to the *Lancet*[1] pointing out the fact of chloroform having been used as an anæsthetic at St. Bartholomew's some months before Sir James's discovery.

"I went out to India again, resumed my duties at the expiration of my furlough, and thought no more about chloroform and its discovery until one day in 1874 I received a letter from Dr. Sanderson, a retired, but formerly eminent member of the Madras Medical Service, enclosing the following communication from Sir R. Christison:—

"'My dear Mr. Sanderson,—I have been trying to meet the tedium of convalescence from a severe influenza by putting together some notes from which I gave, in 1870, a true and particular history of anæsthesia in its several forms. You will see from the enclosed excerpt that a medical officer in your old service is closely connected with the discovery of chloroform anæsthesia, and I think he should be made to put in an appearance, and get what he has a right to. In 1870 I found no Furnell in the Bengal Medical establishment, but in the India List for 1870 I found Michael Cudmore Furnell, surgeon, Madras Army, entered 1855, on furlough. Having no address to direct me, I did not write to him at the time, and afterwards, I fear, forgot the matter till now, when my search after truth has revived.

"'There is no doubt whatever that Lawrence, in the summer of 1847, four or five months before Simpson, used, at Furnell's suggestion, chloroform disguised in the impure state, under the misnomer of chloric ether! *There never was, and there is not now, any such substance. The name put Lawrence and Holmes Coote on a wrong scent.* Had it been called 'spirit of chloroform', which it really was, they would have got at its base in a moment. Now I want you to find out Mr. Furnell for me, and to learn from him where he got his information, and whether he had himself used this miscalled chloric ether. Simpson's investigations were in November of the same year, 1847. I am, yours most truly, R. Christison'.

"I have no copy of my answer to Dr. Sanderson, but it must have been in substance much what I have related in the commencement of this paper. Dr. Druitt, the well-known author of the *Surgeon's Vade Mecum*, was in Madras in 1874, and to him I wrote the letter, in reply to one from him, which appeared subsequently in the *Medical Times and Gazette* of Saturday, May 29th, 1875. The notice of the discovery of chloroform which appeared in that journal, and in which my name is mentioned, owes its existence, no doubt, to his pen.

"Thus matters stood until 1876, when I again came on furlough from India. On my leaving Madras, a paper, the *Madras Standard*, was good enough to publish some complimentary remarks on me, and concluded its notice by mentioning that I was the 'discoverer' of chloroform. To this a correspondent of the *Madras Times*, signing himself X.Y.Z., very properly took exception, pointing out that chloroform was discovered by Soubeiran in 1832; but X.Y.Z. went a step further, and stated 'chloric ether is not chloroform, any more than chloroform is chloric ether.' And again, 'Chloric ether is chloric ether, and chloroform is perchloride of formyle.'

"This letter of X.Y.Z. I first read at my club in London, and it set me thinking if it were possible I had all along been labouring under a mistake about the chloric ether. What was chloric ether exactly? Sir R. Christison, it will be seen, says in his letter, 'There never was, and there is not now, any such substance. The name put Lawrence and Holmes Coote on a wrong scent.' (*vide* extract above), and certainly no such substance is mentioned in our Pharmacopoeia. I determined to solve this matter for my own satisfaction, and accordingly, almost immediately after reading the letter of X.Y.Z., I proceeded to the Pharmaceutical Society's laboratory in Bloomsbury Square, and asked for Professor Redwood, the well-known and eminent chemist. He very kindly explained to me at once exactly what chloric ether was. It was a name synonymous with chloroform, and used also for a spirituous solution of chloroform. (*Vide* Gray's Supplement to the Pharmacopoeia, and Beasley's Pocket Formulary.) For instance we find in Gray's Supplement to the Pharmacopoeia, by Theophilus Redwood, Professor of Pharmacy to the Pharmaceutical Society of Great Britain (published by Longmans and Co., London, 1847), 'Ether chloricus, chloric ether, *chloroform,* terchloride of carbon. These names have been severally applied to a liquid having an etherial (sic) smell, obtained by the distillation of a mixture of weak spirit and chloride of lime' (Dumas). In Beasley's Pocket Formulary we find it thus written:—'Ether chloricus. The so-called medicinal chloric ether is an alcoholic solution of chloroform of variable strength. Mr. Redwood states that what is sold in this country consists of one part of chloroform to six or eight of alcohol.'

"This, of course, at once disposed of X.Y.Z.'s statement that chloric ether and chloroform had no connexion with each other, by demonstrating that they were one and the same thing.

"Sir R. Christison's remark that 'there never was, and there is not now, any such substance', is more difficult to understand. 'There never was any such substance *in the official Pharmacopoeia*' would be intelligible, and is the fact. There is no chloric ether or chloroform mentioned in any of the Pharmacopoeias of that period, 1847. The fact of the matter is that chloric ether or chloroform was very little known at all until Sir James Simpson published an account of its use in 1847, and this, too, is very well shown by Mr. Holmes Coote and Sir William Lawrence's ignorance of what they had got hold of. Even Sir James knew nothing about it until Mr. Waldie, an accomplished pharmaceutist, drew his attention to it. Before 1847 chloroform or chloric ether was a substance very little known, in fact, almost unknown to medical men; it was scarcely a medicinal, but a chemical substance; since that period few substances have become better known in medicine. Nor was the substance chloric ether—*i.e.*, a solution of chloroform in six or eight parts of spirits of wine—a Pharmaceutical preparation; if we look up any of the old Pharmacopoeias we find no mention of it. It was prepared by some eminent chemists of London, such as Bell and Co. of Oxford Street, and Morson, of Southampton Row, and prescribed occasionally as an anodyne by a few eminent practitioners.

"In the present Pharmacopoeia (1867) there is a preparation called spirits of chloroform, of 1 in 18 of spirits of wine, and the reason why it is thus diluted is this. The chloric ether of 1 in 6 has a great tendency, when prescribed in an ordinary mixture, to become disintegrated. The alcohol has a greater affinity for water, and leaves the chloroform, which falls to the bottom. Anyone can easily satisfy himself of this. As I am writing I have on the table before me a small bottle into which has been poured one ounce of chloric ether (1 in 6) and three ounces of water, and then shaken. The chloroform has become separated from the spirit, and lies at the bottom—a thick, oily-looking fluid, very easily distinguished from the supernatant mixture of spirit and water.

"This discovery—for discovery it certainly was to me—that chloroform and chloric ether were names that in 1847 were used for the same substance, very naturally set me thinking whether the bottle I gave Holmes Coote in 1847 was chloroform pure and simple, as described in Gray's Supplement to the Pharmacopoeia, or the alcoholic solution described in Beasley's Formulary. A very simple experiment should determine this. I accordingly wrote to my friend and former fellow-student, Mr. Callender, the well-known surgeon of St. Bartholomew's, and asked him to be good enough, as I had in this country no hospital under my charge, to see if chloric ether—*i.e.*, a solution of chloroform 1 in 6 of spirits of wine—would produce anæsthesia. The following is the result of the experiment, as reported by Mr. Joseph Miles" (this is a mistake for Joseph Mills, the first whole-time anæsthetist at St. Bartholomew's Hospital, appointed in 1875) "the administrator of chloroform at St. Bartholomew's.

"'In compliance with your wish, I have been using the chloric ether—*i.e.*, one part of chloroform and six parts of spirits—for producing anæsthesia during surgical operations. I mixed two fluid ounces of chloroform with ten of alcohol, making a mixture of one part of chloroform to five of alcohol, or one in six; and proceeded to administer it on lint, folded twice (four thicknesses) to the following patients:

"'Case 1.—A woman, aged twenty-four, for the extraction of a toe-nail, was ten minutes getting under the influence, and was kept under ten minutes. There was no reflex action; the anæsthesia was complete.

"'Case 2.—A man, aged forty-seven, for the opening of an abscess, was fifteen minutes getting under the influence, and was kept under seven minutes. Anæsthesia complete.

"'Case 3.—A boy, aged three, for the operation of circumcision, was five minutes getting under the influence, and was kept under ten minutes. Anæsthesia complete.

"' Of the twelve ounces there remains four ounces and two drachms.'

"This very conclusively proves that the dilute chloroform or chloric ether will produce anæsthesia sufficient for all practical purposes, and although it does not prove that the bottle labelled 'chloric ether' first used by Mr. Holmes Coote was not chloroform pure and simple, as I felt after my interview with Professor Redwood at first inclined to think, it shows that there cannot be any doubt that even in its dilute form it can produce anæsthesia, and that Sir R. Christison's statement 'that Lawrence in the summer of 1847, four or five months before Simpson used, at Furnell's suggestion, chloroform (note the curious absence of a comma after the word Simpson, which makes nonsense of the whole argument), disguised in the impure state under the misnomer of chloric ether,' is fully borne out.

"I think Mr. Miles's (Mills's) cases admit of some practical conclusion. Why should not chloroform be always used thus diluted? I think it probable, if it were we should have, few as they are now, fewer accidents. I have always administered chloroform on a handkerchief, in preference to using any machine, from the ease with which in this way we can dilute the anæsthetic with air. It is an expensive but safer way.

"In conclusion, I have only again to reiterate I have written the above lines with no desire whatever, far from it, to detract from the just fame of Sir James Simpson. The fact of my having been the first to use and to introduce the use of chloroform to the profession was made public (with the single exception of the small note in the *Lancet*), not by me but by others, notably by Sir R. Christison; but as the matter has been brought forward, I have felt it would perhaps not be without interest, and it certainly was due to myself and the great school (St. Bartholomew's) of which I was a pupil, to state exactly how it stands. Besides, I must confess it is not without some feeling of pleasure I find my name connected with the discovery of one of the greatest boons ever conferred on suffering humanity." London.

Appendix

To the Editor of the *Medical Times and Gazette*.

"Sir,—Sir Robert Christison, himself in time past a pupil in St. Bartholomew's, has drawn attention to the first use of chloric ether by Sir Wm. Lawrence and Mr. Coote. In the company of my late colleague, Mr. Coote, and my friend, Mr. Furnell, I have heard the facts you allude to more than once narrated, and they are well-known in the school. Perhaps we ought to have published them more widely, but you will find them referred to in the article on Anæsthesia, by Mr. Lister, in the *System of Surgery*, with the exception, which is unfortunately true, of the mention of the intelligence and zeal which prompted Mr. Furnell, whose distinguished Indian career is also well known, to bring chloric ether under the notice of our surgeons, an omission which ought to be remedied in any future edition of the work.

G. W. Callender."

A letter appeared in the next week's *Lancet*[3] which is perhaps worth inserting here:

"Sir,—I have read with much interest, in the *Lancet* of the 30th ult., Dr. Furnell's account of his discovery of the anæsthetic properties of chloric ether —*i.e.*, chloroform diluted with spirit—in the year 1846 (it was, according to Furnell's account, 1847), and I am very glad that he has publicly declared a fact of so much importance, to the knowledge of which he unquestionably has the claim of priority. I feel sure that had Sir James Simpson been living he would have been the first to recognise the claim of the distinguished Indian medical officer, who now so modestly states what ought to have been made better known and fully credited to him long ago. Dr. Furnell says, in reference to certain cases in which spirits of chloroform had been used by Mr. Miles (Mills), 'Why should not chloroform be always used thus diluted?' I would add, why should it not also be generally declared and recognised that the use of chloroform at all as an anæsthetic—one of the greatest boons ever conferred on suffering humanity—is due to the discovery of Dr. M. C. Furnell, of the Madras Medical Service? As he says, 'This would in no way detract from the fame of Sir James Simpson, who (subsequently) made the use of chloroform quickly and widely popular throughout the civilised world,' but who was certainly preceded in the application of the drug as an anæsthetic by an officer who has added many important services during his Indian career to this, the earliest, and perhaps, greatest claim to distinction." J. Fayrer.

Somerset Street, Portman Square, W. July 1st, 1877.

This modest and well-authenticated story is beyond doubt true. In addition to Mr. Coote's evidence and the investigation of Sir Robert Christison, John Snow mentions it in his reply to Syme's lecture on chloroform in 1855. He does not mention Furnell by name, but refers to the incident itself. This shows that the story had been current for about twenty years at the time Furnell wrote his letters. If it had been known, or even suspected, to be false, somebody would surely have written to say so; whereas I did not come across a single letter or quotation of any kind expressing doubt or suspicion.

Furnell's statement that none of the old Pharmacopœias up to 1847 mention chloric ether or chloroform is backed up by Waldie's account of the matter. He had to dispense a prescription containing chloric ether, and had great difficulty in finding any information about it, or how to make it. He finally tracked it down in the United States Dispensatory and was able to prepare some. Owing to the difficulty of obtaining a constant strength he devised a new process, which involved making chloroform itself and then dissolving it in alcohol. And so it happened that, when Simpson asked him if he knew of anything likely to be of use as a substitute for ether, Waldie had the answer ready to hand.

Nineteenth century writers were addicted to an excessive use of commas. Some of their long and involved sentences contain five or six of them, inserted like drawing pins after every word or two, the effect being extremely irritating. Most of them could have been deleted without any loss or change of meaning.

It is curious, therefore, that Furnell, when quoting Christison, omits a very important comma, which changes the whole meaning of the sentence. The more so because Christison's original argument had the comma in its correct place. He said, quite accurately, "There is no doubt whatever that Lawrence, in the summer of 1847, four or five months before Simpson, used, at Furnell's suggestion chloroform. . . ."

Furnell later quotes this as "that Lawrence in the summer of 1847, four or five months before Simpson used, at Furnell's suggestion, chloroform. . . ." It is strange that he should have overlooked this, considering the subject he was writing about, but Furnell's style as a prose-writer was not particularly good.

Holmes Coote's mistake in confusing the Bengal Army and the Madras Army was natural enough. Why should a hospital surgeon, permanently living in England, be expected to know the difference? To Furnell the mistake was important enough to warrant a footnote—but to other people the matter was both unimportant and confusing, all the more so because India and its Government had changed with such bewildering rapidity. When Furnell joined the medical service in India it was under the control of the Honourable East India Company, but when he wrote the letters the Company's sovereignty had departed for ever after the collapse of its authority during the Indian Mutiny. India came under the Crown in 1858. Yet another change took place in 1876, when Victoria became Empress of India; and a more drastic one in 1947, when British rule ended.

Mr. Joseph Mills, who carried out the tests of chloric ether, was merely a chloroformist, and a person of no importance. He was lucky to be mentioned at all, even under the wrong name!

All these little mistakes do not in the least detract from the credibility of the story. If anything they increase it. A person concocting a story which was false would probably take more care to get all his facts correct and his commas in the right places.

References

[1] *Lancet* (1871), Mar. 25. 433.
[2] Sykes, W. S. (1960). *Essays on the First Hundred Years of Anæsthesia.* Vol. I, p. 163. Edinburgh: Livingstone.
[3] *Lancet* (1877), June 30. 934.
Med. Times Lond. (1875), May 29. 587.
(1875), June 5. 617.

CHAPTER 17

A VERY SHORT-LIVED ANÆSTHETIC

INTRAVENOUS anæsthesia began with Oré in 1873, who used chloral. Ether dissolved in saline solution, usually at a strength of 5 per cent., was used to some extent in 1911, notably by Felix Rood.[1] But there was one substance which was used as an intravenous anæsthetic, and so far as I am aware, for nothing else. It only had a short life—nearly all the references to it are compressed into the year 1912; its use must have continued for a short time after this because the Registrar General's figures for anæsthetic deaths from it show one in 1912, two in 1913 and one in 1914. It does not appear in any other years, either before or after these dates.

This substance was hedonal or methyl-propyl-carbinol-urethane. It had the great advantage of pleasantness for the patient, but this was bought at too high a price. In too many cases the pleasant induction was merely a prelude to euthanasia. As far as I can make out there appear to have been 11 deaths from pulmonary œdema in about 1,600 cases.

It had two serious and dangerous faults, which really rendered it quite unsuitable for intravenous use. In the first place it was given in very dilute solution (0·75 per cent.), presumably because of its lack of solubility, so that large quantities of saline were injected with it. One litre or more had to be given during a long operation, which tended to waterlog the patient. In one case the amount given was 1,750 cc. It was also very slowly eliminated, which meant that overdosage was easy and that there was a prolonged period—up to twelve hours—of unconsciousness after the operation. This, of course, increased the risk of pulmonary complications. Not until the easily soluble, rapidly eliminated barbiturates were introduced twenty-one years later did intravenous anæsthesia become the established and popular method which it is today.

Hedonal was first mentioned in the weekly journals on the last day but one of the year 1911.[2] Jeremisch used it in the laboratory, and S. P. Federoff's clinic reported 530 cases from Russia. C. M. Page was one of the first to use it in England.[3] By June, 1912, three deaths had been reported—one from Golden Square Throat Hospital, one from Hull and one in a child of eight in London, who was stated to have status lymphaticus. G. A. H. Barton[4] gave fuller details of the first case a week later. The operation was for a bilateral frontal sinusitis; the post-mortem revealed that the lungs were full of miliary tubercles, and that the trachea and bronchi contained blood. It was thought that the hedonal did not cause death, but contributed to it by depressing the respiration and abolishing the laryngeal reflexes.

Over 300 cases were then reported from the Leeds General Infirmary by R. A. Veale.[5] The pleasant induction was mentioned, but the drug was found to cause thrombosis at the site of injection, local œdema of the dependent lumbar and gluteal regions and, worse still, œdema of the lungs. Three fatal pneumonias occurred in the series. "When 1,100 to 1,200 cc. have been injected the danger zone is entered."

G. A. H. Barton[6] reported 10 cases. He commented on the disadvantage of the prolonged recovery time, and gave some further details of the death which he had previously described. The operation lasted one and a half hours, 1,000 cc. of solution was given, a post-nasal plug was used, and the patient died two hours later without recovering consciousness.

Z. Mennell[7] reported 310 cases from St. Thomas's Hospital, since Mr. Page published his original 200 cases. There had been no death within twelve hours. He considered that excessive doses had been given in the past, and that the skin reflexes should always be brisk. The method had been used in 56 cranial operations.

J. F. Dobson of Leeds[8] recorded 436 cases from February 20th to October 8th with 44 deaths, or 10 per cent. During the same period the general surgical and gynæcological operations totalled 2,302 with 164 deaths, or 7·1 per cent., and out of 1,866 operations with general anæsthesia 120 died, or 6·4 per cent. Of the hedonal patients 5 died from œdema of the lungs, and there were very frequent pulmonary complications.

Mennell wrote again in November.[9] He thought hedonal was contraindicated in operations which caused bleeding into the air passages, in cases of high blood pressure and in cases which could be dealt with safely by other means. Reading between the lines this last phrase appears to mean that Mennell hated the sight of the stuff and thought that it was dangerous. He said that in one case of removal of the tongue for carcinoma the patient died within eight hours, and at the post-mortem a four-inch blood clot was removed from the larynx.

Moynihan said that it gave very good relaxation, better than inhalation anæsthesia.[12]

After this I found no further mention of hedonal. Several outfits for giving it were designed and illustrated, but they did not differ in any important way from ordinary saline infusion apparatus and are not worth illustrating here.

References

[1] *Brit. Med. J.* (1911), Oct. 21. 976.
[2] *Lancet* (1911), Dec. 30. 1847.
[3] *Brit. med. J.* (1912), June 15. 1378.
[4] *Brit. med. J.* (1912), June 22. 1459.
[5] *Brit. med. J.* (1912), Aug. 17. 347.
[6] *Brit. med. J.* (1912), Sept. 14. 612.
Lancet (1912), Nov. 9. 1297.
[7] *Lancet* (1912), Nov. 9. 1297.
[8] *Lancet* (1912), Nov. 9. 1299.
[9] *Brit. med. J.* (1912), Nov. 9. 1311.

Hedonal Apparatus

[10] Felix Rood (1911). *Brit. med. J.*, Oct. 21. 976.
[11] C. M. Page (1912). *Lancet,* May 11. 1258.
[12] B. G. A. Moynihan (later Lord Moynihan) (1912). *Lancet,* June 15. 1631.
[13] W. F. Honan and J. W. Hassler (1913). *Med. Rec. N.Y.,* Feb. 8. 231.
[14] E. G. Schlesinger (1913). *Med. Ann.* 610.
[15] T. T. Higgins (1914). *Lancet,* May 16. 1404.

INDEX

INDEX